The Rape of Emergency Medicine

A Novel By

The Phoenix

The Rape of Emergency Medicine

Published by The Phoenix Publishing Company
P.O. Box 2588
Cambridge, MA 02238-9804

Cover design by Eli Africa

Book production by Comp-Type, Inc., Fort Bragg, CA 95437

Printed in the United States of America

Ordering information. To order additional copies, call or write the distributor:

Mendocino Arts & Gifts
P.O. Box 1063
Mendocino, CA 95460
Phone: (707) 937-3524

ISBN No. 0-9632237-1-2

Library of Congress No. 92-080578

FIRST EDITION

This book is a work of fiction and any resemblance between the characters and real persons, living or dead, is coincidental.

CONTENTS

To

James and Ruth, Jackie and Jeremiah, Robert, Maureen,
Christopher and Peter

PROLOGUE

"...and the Lord hath taken away"
—*Book of Job*

Jenny's body lay on the pathologist's slab. Her tall slender frame belied her mere seven years. It was hard to believe she was so full of life twenty-four hours ago. It was even harder to believe she was such a beautiful girl, now that her body was covered with that hideous, red-blue rash, covered with petechiae *(pa-teek-ee-ii).*

Petechiae are small, 1 to 3 millimeter, oval-round red spots resembling M & M candies. They represent collections of oxygen-carrying red blood cells that have escaped their vessel walls and leaked into the skin. Unlike more benign red rashes, petechiae don't blanch when pressed upon.

Jenny's petechiae were so numerous they coalesced into ecchymotic *(ek-ee-motic)* blemishes. Ecchymosis is the medical term for black and blue marks. Jenny's body was covered from head to toe with little purplish lakes surrounded by innumerable satellites of red spots, sparing only her long blond hair still in a pony tail.

Her mother called the funeral home, but the owner recognized the infectious disease, and told her there was nothing he could possibly do for Jenny now. It would have to be a closed casket with her favorite toys on top. Her mother looked at Jenny for the last time, thinking how much her daughter looked like she'd been beaten, and in fact, Jenny had been beaten—not physically, but by organized emergency medicine.

Paul Adkins was the pathologist on call. He was a brilliant, heavy-set, midwestern farm boy with huge blue eyes and thinning, sandy-blond hair, a muscular former fullback at the University of Illinois at Champaign-Urbana. His loves were biology and the study of disease. He would have stayed in Boston after medical school and residency training had it not been for his other loves, the land and what grew on it.

Not just any land, but Indiana farm land, mid-central Indiana topsoil, eighteen inches deep and so black one always thought it had just rained. It was eighteen inches of fertility where the elongated soybean root, eighteen inches deep itself, enjoyed its finest nurturing home anywhere in the world. Even the Japanese had no trade barriers against these plump little beans, making the world's finest tofu and bean curd. Adkins was harvesting an early crop of soybeans on his father's farm when the call came in. They wanted Jenny autopsied as soon as possible.

Adkins liked to view every body before looking at the medical record. He wanted his own, overall, unbiased impression first. When Adkins first saw Jenny's body, he thought the cause of death to be fulminate Rocky Mountain Spotted Fever. It had been quite some time since he'd seen a body so completely covered with petechiae and ecchymosis. Adkins could already see early, black, gangrenous changes appearing on the tips of Jenny's nose, fingers, and toes. He wondered how she'd caught it so late in the season since he himself hadn't noticed any ticks on the farm dogs in the past month. Rocky Mountain Spotted Fever is spread by the bite of a tick, and is ironically more common in the Midwest than the Rocky Mountains.

Perusing the medical record, he found the diagnosis to be meningitis. This wasn't surprising since meningitis causes a similar dermatologic picture, but with a more rapid demise than Spotted Fever if not recognized and treated early.

At the bottom of the medical record, Adkins noticed something unusual—there were two emergency department charts.

Jenny was seen twice yesterday, within a six hour period, in the emergency room.

The name on the first chart was all too familiar to Adkins. It was Doctor Monk. Monk, as everyone called him, had seen Jenny twenty-four hours earlier. Jenny's mother had brought her in because of cold symptoms, fever, vomiting, and because her daughter "wasn't acting right."

Adkins saw where Monk had noted a rigidity to Jenny's body, a stiff neck being one of the classic signs of meningitis. He saw where Monk had even noted a few peculiar red spots on Jenny's chest. Petechiae are ominous physical findings in any febrile child, demanding an immediate spinal tap and the rapid administration of intravenous antibiotics.

Surely even Monk knew what petechiae were, and most assuredly, Monk could not have seen them, noted them on the medical chart, and not known their significance? Petechiae are red flags waving at even the most unobservant physician shouting meningitis, and spreading petechiae in the presence of a fever grab at the physician demanding intervention.

Meningitis means bacteria growing in the spinal fluid, that rich, nutritious fluid medium that allows intrusive, unwelcomed bacteria to proliferate exponentially. In a matter of hours, the crystal-clear, low-pressure fluid cushioning the brain turns into a turbid, yellow, pus-filled covering that now circumferentially crushes the brain and cranial nerves within the prison of the bony skull. If untreated, the mortality is one hundred per cent, but if recognized and promptly treated, astute clinical physicians can reduce the mortality to less than fifteen per cent. Monk, of course, had not picked up on Jenny's stiff neck, sending her home with a cortisone cream for her rash.

Monk would never see the autopsy report. Earlier that day, Pyramid, Inc., a large emergency medicine physician contract group, called Monk, telling him of their desperate "manpower need" in LaCrosse. One of their emergency physicians had suddenly "taken ill," and the emergency room wasn't "covered" tonight. They told Monk to pick up his tickets at the airport, and they would book the hotel.

Steve Waterbury, the assistant hospital administrator, had tipped off Pyramid, Inc. that Monk had missed another crucial diagnosis, and this one might not blow over so easily.

Adkins, who hated both Waterbury and Pyramid, would surely launch an investigation, and so Norman Lyle, who'd founded Pyramid, Inc. six years ago, took the message himself. He'd become a pro at this, not trusting his junior staff with this type of delicate situation, and actually, this philosophy made Lyle a pretty busy man. Many of the physicians who worked for him had severe problems, but by contracting with many hospitals in various states, he could move bad emergency physicians from place to place until the heat died down. He also thought it best not to tell Monk why he was moved so often. There was no sense discouraging him, and Lyle, instead, improved Monk's morale by telling him he was specially chosen to go to new client hospitals.

Monk would fly to LaCrosse, and Walsh, his replacement, would fly in from Indianapolis. Earlier that week, Walsh was found unarousable while on emergency duty at a Pyramid client hospital. The nurses found an empty bottle of scotch in Walsh's "on call room."

Westerly, Jenny's private family doctor, had recently returned from vacation. He was a good old southern boy who drove a white, nineteen seventy-seven Lincoln Continental still sporting Texas license plates. Westerly was a softly-tailored, charming country doctor, a genteel man with a great big forgiveness pocket who'd been in general medical practice for thirty-five years. He'd just found out about Jenny's death, but Westerly had seen many people die, and he just couldn't understand why Adkins was so angry at that little Monk boy. After all, people with meningitis die and it's that simple. He did wonder why Monk hadn't at least given Jenny some of the latest antibiotic samples the Eli Lilly salesman left in the emergency room. They were free, and it was Monk's trademark to use anything and everything new. Monk's medical professors were the drug salesmen who promoted their new and expensive medicines, telling of the vast number of diseases for which their product was indicated. Good marketing also gave Monk the illusion of being up on the latest medical developments.

"Maybe Monk was slipping?" thought Westerly, who himself, loved to dispense and prescribe medications of all kinds—antibiotics, diuretics, tranquilizers, creams, lotions, salves, anything he felt closest to the patient's needs or potential needs. He loved the look on patients' faces when they were being "treated." They always said "Thank you" when they had a bottle of penicillin in their hands. Westerly was certainly no medical nihilist, having never believed in viruses anyway, or for that matter, any condition for which there was no treatment.

Unfortunately, Doctor Westerly wasn't a very good diagnostician, many of his patients coming back with side effects to the unnecessary medicines. He would then prescribe new medications for their treatment-induced illnesses, making his patients even happier the second time. Patients knew he was brilliant because Westerly was a talkative doctor who always told them in advance of the specific possible side effects, and when his patients came down with their adverse reactions, they were astounded at Doctor Westerly's accuracy. They also felt personally responsible for their side effects because Doctor Westerly had told them, "It only happens to one out of a thousand patients, but you're such a fine person, I'm sure it won't be you." He loved giving his patients their ointments, and they loved rubbing them into their drug-induced rashes.

Ironically, Doctor Westerly had learned a great deal of pharmacology this way. He was a smart man with an impressive memory, and were it not for his laziness, he would have been an excellent clinician as well, but without his vast experience with medical toxicology.

Besides, Westerly enjoyed his reputation, and in fact, local internists occasionally called him, asking his opinion on various medications and their side effects. Once he even opened the monthly County Medical Society meeting with the statement, "I'm not much on diagnosis, but I'm **Hell** on therapy." Even Adkins found himself roaring with laughter. Between Monk's misprescribing and Westerly's overprescribing, the small Indiana farm town of Dupage had become an unknown proving ground for the Food and Drug Administration.

Westerly had to go down to the emergency room to comfort Jenny's family. He also had to give them antibiotics in case they too had become colonized with the meningitis-causing bacteria. The bacteria might be living in their throat or nasal passages since many people carry pathogenic (capable of producing disease) bacteria even though they are not clinically ill.

Eradicating an organism in a nonsymptomatic carrier is a form of prophylaxis. Years ago, Westerly tried to incorporate the word prophylaxis into his working medical vocabulary, but he found it difficult to pronounce and kept getting it confused with immunization.

Westerly gave Jenny's family members some medicines to take for a few days, explaining all the possible side effects.

Westerly, an old-time general practitioner who still "delivered" babies, was suddenly paged to obstetrics. The nurse midwives usually waited until the babies were partially delivered before calling Doctor Westerly since everyone knew it was best if he participated as little as possible in the procedure. He would arrive just as the head and shoulders were delivered, put his hand on the nurse's shoulder, and say, "There,...steady,...a little more to the left,..." and "GOOD," when the legs came out. He would then say very loudly, "I couldn't ah done better myself," and both doctor and mother would share a brief belly laugh. He'd point his finger sternly at the mother, tell her to rest, take plenty of fluids, eat healthy food, and that he would see his brand new patient in two weeks for her first immunization shot. He next prescribed a sleeping pill, told the new mom it might make her dizzy, nauseous, possibly weak, and then left the hospital.

Driving home that afternoon Westerly marveled at how the size of his practice never changed. The number of patients through the years had always remained constant. Jenny was gone, but today the Lord giveth a new life...and a new patient. There was nothing new under the summer sun, even in Dupage.

CHAPTER ONE

STEINERMAN

"Jaundice is the disease that your friends diagnose."
—*Sir William Osler, M.D.*

Abraham David Steinerman was finishing his tenure as the Chief Medical Resident at the Massachusetts General Hospital. He was bittersweetly packing his bags to begin an odyssey, traveling across the country from coast to coast, north to south, his plan being to work along the way in a variety of emergency rooms and health clinics. This was an adventure he'd planned with his wife Shelly for the past five years, and the itinerary included seventeen states, both coasts, two Indian Reservations, and one foreign country to work in a refugee camp. The sojourn would take two years.

Steinerman was careful in his residency to take elective months outside of internal medicine, something quite unusual for today's narrowly-trained specialists. He'd spent months in plastic surgery learning the fine suture techniques for facial lacerations, two months in obstetrics in case of a precipitous emergency room delivery, a trying month in the neonatal intensive care unit, and time in orthopedics perfecting his casting ability, and the difficult x-ray interpretation of pediatric elbow and wrist fractures. He carried a camera at all times, and his slide collection of skin lesions matched that of any of the dermatology residents. His ability to start intravenous lines on drug addicts "with no veins" was legendary, and while in medical school he was a frequent volunteer in the emergency department, becoming an integral part of the trauma team on weekends. He liked surgery, trying to assist on all his own patients, but his intellectual curiosity and fascination for exotic diseases steered him into the specialty of internal medicine as it had his father before him.

Now he was at the pinnacle of his diagnostic acumen. He'd spent an extra year at the General to serve as the Chief Medical Resident where indeed the buck stopped.

Steinerman was a true physician, the kind all patients would ask for if they only knew how to access such information. He ran the medical service of the Massachusetts General at an exciting time, being at the forefront of elucidating many new diseases including toxic shock syndrome and Legionnaire's disease. He was one of the first to connect the rare Kaposi's skin cancers and the highly unusual pneumocystis pneumonia with homosexual young men. He and his father had long noted the increased incidence of teenage arthritis at the General, readily implementing the advice from the Yale group on Lyme disease. He didn't believe in the herpes scare, predicted "the epidemic" would never materialize, and watched the hoopla slowly die down after *Time* magazine's sensational stories. Steinerman had, in his four years of residency training, seen every disease, except one, described in the most widely read and respected textbook, *Harrison's Principles and Practice of Internal Medicine.*

When Steinerman was up and awake, no one dared to sleep, and more importantly, no one ever dared to refuse to come in, even in the wee hours of the morning. The radiologists, pathologists, surgeons and anesthesiologists knew when Steinerman was on call, and even the dermatologists knew his schedule. When a patient came to the Massachusetts General needing a rapid diagnosis, there was no limit to Steinerman's evaluation. Biopsies were done and the pathologists were called in at three a.m. to fix and stain and read the slides *that night,* radiology residents were called to tomography scan, resonance scan, and angiogram *that night,* hematologists were called to examine bone marrows, pulmonary to interpret function studies, gastroenterology to pinpoint the exact locus of any stomach or colon bleed—everyone *that night.* During Steinerman's tenure, the sun never rose at the Massachusetts General on an undiagnosed patient, and unlike many who preceded him, Steinerman's residents, interns, medical students, nurses, and even the hourly-paid, overworked technicians enjoyed working with him. They loved his judgment, his meticulous and precise diagnostic style, and they particularly enjoyed his assessment and intervention in a life-threatening illness. They enjoyed being part of his team, everything it was and represented, and in fact, they loved Steinerman.

But now it was time to leave. After Shelly's death he had immersed himself in internal medicine. The first year internship, the scourge of a medical doctor's life, actually gave Steinerman a structured existence. He could stay up all night returning home only to sleep. In the empty house, alone he would sleep, thankful to return the next day to stay up another thirty-six straight hours, thirty-six hours of hell for the other twenty-two medical interns, but a welcome refuge for Abraham Steinerman.

Shelly Wiener and Steinerman were in the same medical school class and married in their first year. Their first summer of medical school they spent together, volunteers in an Israeli hospital, working all day, eating outdoors, drinking red wine in the warm summer evenings by the Mediterranean Sea and making love at night in their small cozy apartment. It marked his happiest days, and he never thought the romantic high of their lives could ever end, but now he blamed himself for Shelly's death, for he'd stayed in the same state of denial she did. Neither one mentioned the excessive amount of bleeding when she brushed her teeth. "We'll have to go to the dentist for some cleaning when we have time. I'll pick up some floss on my way home." Shelly, a vivacious energetic woman, started to take naps. "It's medical school, it's just so fatiguing." There they were, a *folie à deux,* a true psychiatric pair, staying blissfully unaware. It was their friend, Philip Mahoney, who first sat them down, and "broke the news" that Shelly was visibly jaundiced. Her subsequent death was rapid and Steinerman, the budding internist, never forgave himself. He would get up in the morning and carve out a slice of guilt for himself, a generous slice.

Philip Mahoney told him though, he and Shelly had actually become one, and one person doesn't diagnose jaundice. Mahoney also reminded him, "Besides, Shelly was spared the General's death. It would have been a death preceded by a Nagasaki dose of radiation, medications to stimulate her nausea center twenty-four hours a day, slough her skin and cripple her mind, and all for a few extra weeks of life—no, not real life, existence. Come on Abe, you know Shelly. She had a few extra weeks of *arbeiten und lieben* and that's the way we all would have wanted it."

Shelly was an unusual woman, and it was true, that's the way she would have wanted it, but Steinerman had fallen in love only once in his life, and knew it was unlikely ever to happen again with this intensity. He was sad, more sad than depressed, but despondently sad. All who knew Shelly felt at the time Steinerman was probably right, but rather than the alcohol Mahoney and most of the residents would have chosen, he sought out a different addiction, work, and the internship and residency in internal medicine were a perfect fix. He was abused by the other residents, and given an inordinate amount of "unit time" in his first two years. Mostly he was assigned to the arduous intensive care unit rather than the more observational coronary care unit, but that was another man's hell, it was Steinerman's escape.

All his closest friends had left Boston after medical school. He'd been with Mahoney through Boston Latin, Brown undergraduate, and Harvard med, but now Mahoney was gone, gone to the Hershey Medical Center in Pennsylvania to begin a residency in this new medical specialty called emergency medicine. Shelly was gone, and Steinerman was alone on the desolate floors of the battle-scarred General—alone to stay up all night, alone in Boston through its uninhabitable winters. It was literally a depraved life, enclosed by the Lysol-scented, paint-chipped walls of the General's medical wards, the dormitories where any patient younger than seventy-three was considered pediatrics, a craven, structured existence for Steinerman, and thank God it was available to him.

But one couldn't always be a medical resident, one couldn't smolder in grief and guilt and lead a structured life forever. It was time to go. He was offered a fellowship in cardiology, but that would mean more structured time and work, more of the fix he craved. Mahoney finally had to tell him, "It's time to go, Abe." It was time to leave the General, and time to leave Massachusetts.

Abraham David Steinerman's first interaction with organized emergency medicine was the signing of a contract with Pyramid, Inc.

CHAPTER TWO

THE CONTRACTS AND THEIR HOLDERS

"As through this world I ramble.
I see lots of funny men;
Some will rob you with a six gun,
Some with a fountain pen."
—*Woody Guthrie*

Norman Lyle didn't notice Steinerman enter because Lyle was completely absorbed in the major task of all emergency medicine "management" groups—filling in the blanks.

A "blank" is a well known term in the field of emergency medicine. Every month a set of twelve hour "blanks" has to be "filled in" for every basic emergency room in the country. Each month a set of blank squares is printed up for each client hospital of so called "management" groups. The set of blanks is actually nothing more than a simple calendar, a set of blocks, thirty-one days to fill in, and thirty-one nights to fill in. All sixty-two blanks of the calendar have to be filled in with the name of a physician agreeing to "cover."

Lyle was quite busy as Pyramid, Inc. had many hospital contracts in many states with many blanks to fill in. He always worked on the initial set of blanks for a new client hospital himself. It was imperative that physicians like Monk and Walsh not be allowed in hospitals until Pyramid, Inc. passed the sixty-day probation period. Lyle was lucky this month because Bing, one of the all time best "start-up-physicians" for new client hospitals, was available.

Bing was in Lyle's office, and Lyle had Bing penciled into the blank squares at least fourteen times this month at two different hospitals. Lyle looked at the daily census figures from the new hospital contracts trying to schedule Bing at the busiest periods, Friday night, Saturday night, etc.

Also, it was essential to have Bing back in on Monday mornings. Just in case any of the docs filling in other blanks messed up over the weekend—and they usually did—Bing could put out the brush fires, especially in those sensitive beginnings. Monday mornings were well-known trouble spots to experienced group "managers" in emergency medicine.

Steinerman was equally immersed, looking out over the soothing boat traffic in the Boston Harbor and the breathtaking, expansive views from Pyramid's office. Not even the neurosurgeons had posh citadels this lavish with such panoramic views.

"Lyle must do something other than 'fill in the blanks?'" wondered Steinerman. He noticed his name printed on the daily bulletin board, "Welcome Doctor Steinerman!" Suddenly he was greeted by one of the well-dressed administrative assistants, Alex C. Patterson.

"You must be Doctor Steinerman. Can I get you some coffee? Doctor Lyle is in with Doctor Bing, but they should be finished any minute. They're just working on next month's blanks, uh..., I mean schedules."

"Nice to meet you. No thanks on the coffee, Alex. I'm all coffeed out."

"Well just make yourself at home. We're all like one big family here, you know. I have to run and return a phone call to our Chicago office."

"Your Chicago office?"

"Yes, Doctor Steinerman, we also have branch offices in Dallas and Jacksonville, and we're just opening a new office in

Los Angeles. Again, Doctor, please let us know if there's anything you need."

"Thanks, Alex."

Looking inward through the floor-to-ceiling glass doors, Steinerman stared at the main ingredient of any emergency medicine "management" group, the telephone banks, all manned with young, energetic boys and girls. They were in a gymnasium-sized area, at least twenty-five of them, all yacking as hard as they could on the phone. Every one of them had a set of calendar blocks, a set of blanks they were filling in for Pyramid's numerous client hospitals. They were each constantly turning through several Rolodexes of names and phone numbers, the whole scenario looking like a public broadcasting station during pledge week.

"But who were they calling?" Steinerman wondered. The young enthusiastic boys and girls on the phones with blanks and Rolodexes were known in emergency medicine parlance as "pledge drivers." What Steinerman didn't know was the boiler rooms in Dallas, Los Angeles, Jacksonville, and Chicago were also buzzing like beehives with whole cadres of these unskilled laborers "filling in the blanks" to "cover" the emergency rooms throughout the nation.

"But who were the pledge drivers calling?" Steinerman wondered.

As a matter of fact, most of the physicians filling in the blanks were unskilled labor themselves. Very few of these physicians had been to boot camp to learn basic skills, virtually none of them having any formal emergency medical training. The boys and girls on the phones never asked because if they could contact a physician with a current, unrevoked, state medical license then a blank was legally filled. That was their job, "to fill in the blanks," by making entries on the calendar blocks with the names of physicians from the Rolodexes.

When these deputized physicians showed up for roll call at the hospital for their twelve or twenty-four hour shifts, they were promptly given battlefield commissions, and became known as "the emergency room doctors." Pledge drivers "filling in the blanks" represented the heart and soul of large and small emergency medicine "management" groups.

By nineteen-eighty, Pyramid, Inc. had become a blank-filler operation of Biblical proportions, with nothing even remotely resembling this existing in any other field of medicine. There were no pledge drives seeking orthopedists, no blanks to fill in in radiology, no unskilled laborers working a day or two in obstetrical practices or Hollywood Squares of surgery.

"Surely someone keeps tabs on all of this?" thought Steinerman in those first few minutes, and "it must be that so-called American Academy of Emergency Physicians that Philip Mahoney mentioned. But don't they..."

Suddenly Lyle came out with Doctor Bing who quickly greeted Steinerman. Lyle introduced himself, but Doctor Bing needed no introduction to the Steinerman family.

"How are you Doctor Bing? My father mentioned you'd left your obstetrical practice to do emergency medicine," said Steinerman politely.

Bing said, "Yes, and I hear you're coming on board with Pyramid. Let me know if there's anything you need. We're all like family here." Bing mentioned that he was in a rush, seemed mildly uncomfortable, and quickly left.

Lyle was impressed, as was everyone, with Steinerman's appearance and demeanor, and in fact, Lyle remembered the Steinermans from his old neighborhood. Steinerman was tall and elegant, and his manner was self-assured, confident, but not in any way cocky. As he told Lyle of his two-year plan, Lyle assured him he had come to the best possible "management" group to map his odyssey, explaining, "The family of Pyramid is growing. We'll soon be in all fifty states and possibly other countries one day. In fact, we're expanding operations at an explosive rate, and many hospitals throughout the country are calling daily for Pyramid's valuable 'services.' "

"Pyramid's 'services,' " Steinerman wondered, "What are

the 'services?' Filling in the blanks is surely just a minor part of this incredible operation, isn't it?"

Ironically Steinerman liked Lyle, and would later continue to admire his discipline and intense drive. Somehow Lyle would maintain his thin, classy appearance throughout all those rich luncheons and dinners with hospital administrators replete with Beluga and Dom Perignon. Steinerman would chuckle about this in later years—Lyle, *The Thin Man,* still up in that office, tirelessly filling in the blanks while the human waves of Steinermans, Mahoneys, Monks, Walshes, and a cast of thousands saw the patients in the emergency rooms of the nation.

Steinerman noticed some unusual clauses in the contract Lyle asked him to sign, lots of paragraphs he'd never noticed in other branches of medicine. Things like:

> "The physician shall in no way speak or write to officers of any Pyramid, Inc. client hospital about anything that might result in the loss of income to the company."

"Standard," said Lyle, trying to talk inconsequentially.

> "...the physician, hereinafter referred to as the subcontractor, shall disclose no proprietary information..."

"There are copycats out there. They're not up to our quality, and the disclosure of trade secrets might jeopardize our position. We have a duty to our client hospitals," Lyle explained.

"What in the world was proprietary information? What are trade secrets in emergency medicine, and why all the restrictive language?" Steinerman knew of no trade secrets in internal medicine, and those words, proprietary information, trade secrets, and above all, "quality," seemed to be getting a lot of (over)use as Steinerman read on,

> "The company shall charge a rental fee of fifteen dollars per twelve hour shift for the use of books, articles, and various appliances purchased by the company and used by the subcontractors."

"Tax reasons," replied the poker face Lyle. "It's common

practice to charge a facility fee. Of course, we don't actually charge the fee, but if the right people ask, we just tell them it's already been taken out of your agreed upon subcontracting fee." Lyle picked up on Steinerman's wariness, and looking aggrieved, he said, "You see, Doctor Steinerman, we take care of the business so you can practice medicine."

"The right people," Steinerman continued to wonder, "who are they and what do they ask?"

Steinerman vaguely remembered the Lyle family from South Boston, but didn't recall they'd received a great inheritance or won the Irish Sweepstakes. As Steinerman saw Lyle presiding over a vast fortune, he was reminded of that quote from Balzac, "Behind every great fortune, there is a crime."

Lyle had to leave the office for ten minutes to make copies of the contract, and Steinerman used Lyle's phone to quietly call Philip Mahoney, who was working in a nearby emergency room, to ask about the "crime."

"Philip, who are these people? I think there's something unwholesome going on up here. I think there are a few weeds in this garden called emergency medicine."

"Actually, Abe, the Pyramid is more like Agent Orange being dropped on the landscape of emergency medicine."

"Are they specialists in emergency medicine?"

"They're subspecialists in their own field, highway robbery."

"Why do these operations exist, Philip?"

"We haven't got any pesticide that works on them yet," Mahoney laughingly replied. "It's a big racket, Abe. We'll talk about it later. I'll fill you in. It's a good story. Gotta go for now, the E.R. is swamped. By the way, how did you like 'Norman's Kids.' "

"Norman's Kids?"

"That's what we call all those young kids up there on the phones. Cecil Grimes once said Pyramid's office looks like a Jerry Lewis telethon, so we call them Norman's Kids."

"Philip, wait, wait one minute. What about the Academy?"

"You mean the thumbs up their asses?"

"The thumbs up their asses?"

"Yes, the ranking members of the Academy put their thumbs up their asses whenever the issue of Pyramid comes up. They sit in their new office building right across the street from Lyle's satellite office with their thumbs up their asses. It's what they do best," as Mahoney's voice turned sarcastic. "We'll talk about it later. This place is beginning to back up, and I've got two ambulances on the way."

"Wait one more minute, Philip. Just tell me how much money they make."

"The toll collectors take in between ten and twenty-five thousand dollars a month clear profit per hospital they manage."

"Whaaat! A month? Philip, they must be working on at least twenty hospitals up there. You can't be..."

"Abe, I've got to go, got to go, got a full house. We'll talk all about it later."

Lyle slipped with Steinerman. He could usually pick out a potential troublemaker who fit the profile early on, but his impression of this well-spoken, brilliant physician touched even Lyle, a kind of vestigial physician himself, useless but remnant, and capable, like the appendix, of causing trouble even to the death of the organism. Lyle would grow to battle this tall, wiry, good-looking chief resident from the General, but he would always clearly remember that first hour interview with Abraham David Steinerman. Lyle told his wife to contact Steinerman if he or any member of the family became ill.

But Lyle usually avoided the Steinermans, normally keeping their type off the reservation, physicians who asked too many questions about insurance policies and tail coverage (insurance coverage after a physician left the group), or pried into billings or any other matters the clinical emergency physician wasn't supposed to know about. Curious, bright physicians like Steinerman would pick up early on the scam, pointing out the emperor's lack of clothes, and unlike Mahoney, they weren't dreamers, and might speak to the "wrong" people. Fortunately, even if they did, there was no one to speak to. The American Academy of Emergency Physicians saw to that.

Steinerman inked the many-layered and well-lawyered contract in the palatial offices of Pyramid, Inc., high in the John Hancock Building, and felt the journey was about to begin. He tried to contact his old Harvard Medical School friend, Paul Adkins, to tell him of his upcoming trip to Dupage, Indiana, but Adkins was at the regional midwestern meeting of the American Academy of Pathologists.

Adkins was in the company of a dozen pathologists when, to his surprise, the pathology group started telling Doctor Monk stories. How did they all know Monk?

Pyramid, Inc. held many emergency room "management" contracts in the midcentral states, and Monk was routinely scheduled around to dilute his presence at any one client hospital. The pathologists laughed at this Gypsy doctor Pyramid used to "fill in the blanks" of its emergency room schedules over a five state region. Adkins laughed, pointing out Monk was more of a serial killer than a Gypsy doctor, and they all roared with laughter while exchanging autopsy stories.

Adkins had a lingering sense of ill ease on the drive home remembering the countless stories of Pyramid's troubled physicians, that Rolodex collection of drunks, incompetents, "recovering" addicts, rheumatoid neurosurgeons, pathologic liars, paranoids, schizoids, "retired" surgeons, and sociopaths cashiered out of other specialties. He remembered Jenny's autopsy and the condition of her brain. The human brain should have mountains and deep canyons running through it called gyri and sulci. Jenny's brain was so swollen, it lacked any landmarks, no gyri or sulci, just flat as a pancake from all the pus and bacteria pushing her grey matter unmercifully against the unyielding bony vault of her skull. Adkins had always viewed Monk as actively homicidal in the emergency room, but Pyramid, Inc. had made a quantum leap, bestowing a genocidal influence over the heartland.

Adkins continued to be disturbed by the thought of large "management" groups shifting emergency room doctors from hospital to hospital over whole regions of the nation. Surely the American Academy of Emergency Physicians knew of these scurrilous practices, and had written guidelines to reign in the unbridled growth of these profiteers?

The next morning Adkins called the Academy, explaining his concern, and was transferred to Goldman, the spokesperson of the Academy for business and ethical matters.

Adkins didn't know at the time Goldman owned over twenty-five very-lucrative, east-coast emergency room "management" contracts, making over one-hundred-and-eighty-thousand-dollars profit per year per contract, and had used both Monk and Walsh in the past. Goldman had also just secured a new contract to provide staff to an emergency room, and, in fact, was expecting to use both Monk and Walsh to fill in the imperative "blanks."

Goldman explained to Adkins the contract holders had invested their own money in the formation of these groups, and by putting their money at risk were entitled to reap the harvest. After all, this was the basis of capitalism, and as the "chief executive officer" of a "small business," he knew first-hand the perils of risk.

Adkins was slightly nauseated at Goldman's smugness, and angered by his simple-minded business presentation. He almost burst out laughing when Goldman told him the Constitution itself might crumble if the unfettered growth of the multistate emergency medicine "management" groups was tampered with.

But hadn't Goldman heard the learned professions were regulated since their inception? Multistate emergency medicine "management" groups, somewhat dubious entities at best, corporate emergency-medical-care providers didn't require special forms of regulation?

Adkins rather accurately visualized Goldman as a well-dressed, balding, overweight endomorph with his lips locked in a persistent half-smile. Goldman went into a near babble, explaining the basis of all medical growth was like everything else, determined by the marketplace.

"The marketplace? Like the silver market?" asked Adkins.

"Exactly!" cried Goldman deliriously, continuing on with his preposterous self-serving crock of shit.

All of a sudden it hit Adkins. No, it couldn't be? The quality of emergency care for a sixteen-year-old high-school football player with a fractured neck was determined by the marketplace? The elderly with fractured hips and congestive heart failure, a young family man with an acute brain hemorrhage—their emergency care all determined by the marketplace? Adkins chilled as a sudden horror iced his spinal cord into a numbing paralytic daze. Every neuron in his head was silenced. His body turned pale. He was soaked in his own cold sweat. For the first time in his life he experienced *the horror,* one of those passages of maturity he now wanted to retreat from. He wasn't writing an essay about it, seeing it, or reading about it, but experiencing the *horror* as Adkins realized the diagnosis of meningitis in a seven-year-old girl was determined by the marketplace, and not just any marketplace, but one completely without morals or regulations, fashioned out of physician and patient deception, one of mindless compulsive greed, Goldman's marketplace, Pyramid's marketplace, and above all, the American Academy of Emergency Physicians' marketplace.

After thirty-five minutes of Goldman, Adkins hung up. He had trouble laying the telephone receiver into its cradle. His hands were trembling with rage.

CHAPTER THREE

SUITS AND SCRUBS

"In the beginning..."
—*Genesis*

Norman Lyle could be summed up in one phrase, he was a nice guy—a tall, thin, richly-spoken executive carrying himself particularly well in an expensive suit, effortlessly exuding a certain aristocratic air.

Lyle was born, though, with a comparative disadvantage, a perceived disadvantage, for in Boston, several blocks of real estate determined one's social strata, and once one was branded, certain upward movements were impossible. One couldn't be a Daughter of the American Revolution without having a mother who was the daughter of one. The so-called blue bloods kept a very limited access to their club, and Norman Lyle intensely disliked the thought of not belonging with the Lowells, Cabots, and Lodges.

As a child Norman lived in a middle-class arena in view of the Beacon Hill estates, the area where he desperately wished to be living. Although it was not Hampton Court and Washington never slept there, his home was a substantial middle-middle class house with a full basement and front and back yards.

But somewhere early on, the young Lyle got hooked on this Royalty thing, and through his bedroom window he could see the cupolas and turrets of one particular home, fixating his peculiar frustration, the sense of not belonging, on this, the grandest of the Hill's noble homes, the Doctor Francis Peabody estate.

Just outside of Beacon Hill where blue-blooded WASPdom ended, a more recent layer of human evolution displayed itself—a lower to mid-middle class area just short of Roxbury where much of the comparative disadvantage could be credited to alcohol. Perhaps it was not always a pretty sight, and certainly the Irish, Italian, and Jewish neighborhoods of the south end of Boston cast into suspicion the notion that all God's children are beautiful. But even in their less attractive moments, there always existed a strong, working-class spirit in Boston, and it was indeed an upwardly mobile area, much of it credited to the Massachusetts public school system of the nineteen fifties and sixties culminating in the crown jewel of American education, the Boston Latin School, where the learning of both Latin and Greek were basic four-year requirements of continued attendance.

The Boston Latin School offered a cultural and intellectual milieu launching an inordinate number of immigrant children into extraordinarily productive lives, making many a fairy tale come true. The students received a classical humanist education with a firm understanding of antiquity while becoming well versed in invertebrate zoology and Maxwell's equations if not Unified Field Theory. There were no intellectual limitations at the Boston Latin School, and many of the blue bloods sent their children to Boston Latin rather than the Phillips Exeter or Andover Academies, enjoying the fact their children lived with the rich but played with the poor, and Latin and Greek speaking poor to boot. *Only in America.*

During the late sixties, the spineless "managers" of the Latin School gradually let these curriculum requirements of formal education lapse, promptly blaming it on the rising black population. The blue bloods stopped sending their children to Boston Latin when the Latin and Greek requirements were loosened, also blaming it on the blacks.

In an odd way, the non-immigrant rich are still different, for there are no Doctors Rockefeller or Surgeons Vanderbilt in America. There are no Whitneys or Mellons in the field of medicine, and it was the rather precocious Norman Lyle, an above average but not overbright student at the Latin, who sensed this biodata early on. The very rich in America don't become physicians, and this Maginot line of education is rarely if ever crossed. The days of the aristocratic Doctors Francis Peabody and Paul Dudley White ended for no apparent reason, all wealthy American dynasties sending their children to law school instead, to law school to learn how the world works, law schools like Harvard, Yale, New York University, Georgetown, or the University of Virginia at Charlottesville.

The only barbaric educational institution that no one from the Latin or from Boston, whether rich or poor, ever attended was the vile Johns Hopkins University. But the fact remains among American doctors, there are no latter-day blue-blooded physicians, only new names like Debakey, Wong, and Fauci, along with another list resembling an Israeli phonebook. Norman Lyle wasn't a Jew, he wasn't Irish or Italian, he wasn't a Roman Catholic, but a proper Protestant albeit a commoner, living a few mean blocks west of Beacon Hill. His family was not poor, offering Norman sufficient latitude to choose his career, but Lyle never did explain to anyone why he eventually went to medical school instead of law or government school, especially after acquiring the necessary insights to lead his chosen life. He graduated from the Latin, Brown University, spent a year at Yale Divinity, and then surprised everyone by going to medical school.

Of course, the title "doctor" pretty much summed up everything anyone ever hoped for in those days, "doctor" being more than sufficiently uppercrust. It is still unknown to this day why Norman Lyle was so conscious of class distinctions, particularly the family genealogies, the aristocratic eccentricities, and all that *Mayflower* caboodle. These were certainly unimportant notions to non-Anglophiles growing up in the Colonies in the nineteen fifties and sixties.

In fact, most New Englanders simply viewed the British as a group with an annoying set of mannerisms that got their ass kicked on Bunker Hill. But Norman J. Lyle for very obscure reasons to everyone, never seemed to fit, or at least somewhere deep in the recesses of his psyche, he felt that he never fit.

After finishing a rotating internship, Norman got his first job as the company doctor at the corn flakes factory. He did pre-employment physicals, took care of sprained ankles and sore throats, sutured minor lacerations, and pretty much languished in his role as the company "doc." Occasionally he got a seriously burned patient from the sugar frosted flakes building where employees sometimes got hot sugar burns since the sugar had to be heated to two hundred degrees into a hot syrup in order to be sprayed onto the corn flakes. Working with the frosted flakes was a much more dangerous job than working with corn flakes, and the insidious progression of the hot syrup burns did interest Lyle somewhat. But the burns were infrequent, and Lyle spent long days listening to the employees' endless complaints of lower back pains, chronic fatigue syndromes, and depression. His left-sided migraines, which hadn't recurred since neuroanatomy classes, were reactivated.

Lyle continuously sent away for brochures on various residency programs to formalize the continuance of his medical education, but no field of medicine interested him enough to complete three more years of residency training. Lyle knew all along he didn't fit into the world of clinical medicine, but on weekends he would work a night or two in a local Boston emergency room. He hoped the emergency room's broad exposure to all sub-specialities in all age groups would give him an interest, a direction, a niche, a medical specialty he could devote his life to, a place where he could fit in. Lyle didn't dislike emergency medicine, and he did very much enjoy wearing the clothing of the nighttime doctor, the matching top and bottom, loosely fitting, pajama-like surgical garb referred to as "scrubs." It resembled a uniform, reminding him of his first little-league outfit, and he liked being called one of the "scrubs," the "scrubs" being a nickname for those physicians who actually saw, evaluated, and treated sick and injured patients.

Besides, Lyle made twenty dollars an hour working in his field of dreams as a "scrub," giving him an extra few hundred bucks every week to play with, quite a tidy sum in those days.

It so happened in the early nineteen seventies, at a low point in Lyle's drifting life, the hospital administrator at Saint Ann's Hospital in South Chelsea asked Norman if he had a friend who might be interested in working Tuesday or Friday nights in the emergency room. The semi-purposeless Lyle said "probably," and late one afternoon he called some of his classmates who were completing residencies in internal medicine or general surgery to see if they could work a few nights a month to staff the emergency room at Saint Ann's. A few of them said they had some spare time, and asked Lyle how much money it paid.

Norman Lyle answered with something incomparably unpremeditated, something that was about to change forever the face, the concept, the philosophy, the structure, the field, the nature of the discipline called emergency medicine as Norman Lyle said, "It pays fifteen dollars an hour." Instead of twenty dollars an hour, the job suddenly paid fifteen an hour. Lyle never knew what in the spur of that devilish moment made him say fifteen instead of twenty or even eighteen or nineteen an hour. Without any conscious consideration, without even the vaguest notion of a profit-and-loss balance sheet, and certainly with no malice aforethought, the ill-fitting Norman Joseph Lyle, sitting there on the counter in the sugar frosted flakes building, set into motion the genesis of the largest covert health care swindle in the history of American medicine.

All of the resident yeomen agreed to work, and before long, Lyle had filled in a set of names on the blank calendar for the hospital administrator, and not just Tuesday and Friday, but every night and weekends.

But the young Lyle sat there in fear. "Five bucks an hour—that's twenty-five per cent just for scheduling them. What if I get caught?" Sitting there dressed in his working "scrubs" Lyle re-thought, "Heck, they'll just view it as another school-boy prank if they find out. Maybe they'll make me give it back, or maybe they'll even let me keep a buck or two an hour for scheduling. It's good money, certainly worth a try."

Little did Norman Lyle know how far back into the future he'd just stepped. How could Norman have possibly realized that little snowball he started rolling could grow so big when setting the twenty-five per cent of gross revenue commission for scheduling other physicians to see, evaluate, and treat emergency patients in Massachusetts.

Lyle's only request was that the hospital administrator pay Lyle directly, and he would distribute the monies to the residents. Lyle requested this out of fear the administrator might find out how much the scheduling fee was, the unknowing Lyle setting into motion yet another industry standard of emergency medicine scheduling, secrecy, the utmost of secrecy, little secrets mixed with a few small lies, eventually becoming known as "proprietary information."

The hospital administrator in South Chelsea was impressed, though, particularly since the emergency department was becoming more of a demanding headache in the early seventies, especially with those motorcycle accidents, those rape patients now called victims, those beat-up kids renamed battered children, and the damn investigational five o'clock news broadcast.

He also felt Lyle did him a second favor by taking care of the payroll of the emergency-room doctors as well. So the hospital administrator breathed a sigh of relief, and Norman Lyle was suddenly making five dollars an hour for scheduling the residents of Boston to work in the local emergency room in their spare time.

Five dollars an hour might not seem like much, but Lyle

scheduled twelve hours every night during the week (the local physicians rotated call without reimbursement during the day) and twenty-four hours a day on Saturdays and Sundays. Lyle worked exactly one hour a day during his lunch break to schedule one month of coverage, making just about as much money as he did in the frosted flakes factory, so he quit. He quickly obtained a second hospital to schedule, then a third and even a fourth. He was making a handsome sum for just about an hour's work a day per hospital. But even more than the money, Norman Lyle began to feel something, a great stirring deep within himself, an almost ancestral sense of peace when he suddenly realized he was beginning to fit.

Lyle's wife Carolyn, the former Carolyn Skanks, helped her husband with the scheduling. Before they'd had their first child, Carolyn held a daytime job with a fly-by-night outfit providing private security guards for hospitals, museums, and school playgrounds. The firm operated without a terribly wide margin of safety, having many citizens with less than impeccable credentials employed as security guards.

Carolyn helped Norman because she found the job of scheduling doctors to work in the emergency rooms remarkably similar to her daytime job in the contract security-guard industry.

Both the positions of security guards and emergency-room doctors did require applicants to be screened, making sure they were not undocumented aliens nor in possession of any recent felony convictions, and in the case of the doctors, they also had to possess a current, unrevoked, Massachusetts medical license.

The former Carolyn Skanks began to know most of the medical and surgical residents of Boston by name, noting the rapid turnover in both of her scheduling jobs. She also screened out the rather obnoxious physicians who asked to be paid more money—the old rate before Lyle started taking his twenty-five per cent cut—especially for the busier night and weekend shifts. Carolyn tried not to use them because she and

Norman wanted to employ doctors and security guards at the lowest competitive bid, even though it always seemed to be the more substantial, but snappier doctors who asked for more money. Norman and the former Carolyn Skanks realized early on they would rather cut corners, and deal with complaining hospital administrators, making more money themselves, than hire the best doctors in Boston. Because of this stratagem, Norman Lyle fancied himself "a good businessman." After all, he and Carolyn had a baby on the way, and housing prices in Massachusetts were still going up in the seventies.

One day, Carolyn brought two Rolodexes from an office supply store to keep all the names in order, and to have a method of adding new names and clearing out the names of physicians and security guards who'd moved or decided not to work for them any more. In time, Carolyn quit her difficult daytime job because scheduling security officers required her to kick the tires occasionally, but randomly scheduling emergency physicians was totally unregulated, and paid so much more. The former Carolyn Skanks marveled at the concept of the Rolodex, an ingenious creation, a tool perfectly fitted to help fill in the blanks of emergency room schedules.

Little could the former Carolyn Skanks have known, sitting there in 1971, in her kitchen, what lavish Rolexes those innocent little Rolodexes would generate in the years to come. She and Norman liked filling in the blanks of the schedules from the table in their kitchen, and they became the first of the "kitchen schedulers" of emergency medicine.

Carolyn very much liked having Norman around on weekends, enjoying his new found enthusiasm. She was glad he was out of the corn flakes factory and underneath, she was relieved he was out of clinical medicine altogether, but Norman Lyle and the former Carolyn Skanks were releasing a movement from their otherwise sensible kitchen that was to have epic consequences on organized emergency medicine.

Every week, Lyle promptly picked up his kitchen scheduling check from the hospital administrator's office. He felt quite savvy, depositing the check into one of the new interest-bearing checking accounts from which he paid the residents monthly, thereby earning a few kopeks of interest in the meantime. This little maneuver, suggested by the bank's vice president, again made Lyle fancy himself "a good businessman."

Walking by the entrance to the emergency room one day, Lyle noticed a new ambulance, in fact, a new type of ambulance vehicle.

For literally generations, ambulances were Cadillacs, white Cadillacs that brought patients from their homes and accident scenes to the hospitals. Lyle remembered the white Cadillac that picked up his dying grandfather, taking him to the "accident room," the old name for the emergency department.

White Cadillacs that could carry a patient in the supine position were an integral part of the American landscape in the nineteen sixties and early seventies. They contained very few pieces of equipment, maybe a splint or two, and a small *Johnson & Johnson* first aid box. Black Cadillacs bringing patients from the hospital to the funeral home, and from the funeral home to the cemetery, were the same makes and models as the white ones, and curiously enough, usually owned and run by the same funeral homes. There was no conflict of interest since the patients in the white Cadillacs usually ended up in the black Cadillacs after their ordeal in the "accident room."

The transition from the white Cadillac to the black Cadillac was pretty much taken for granted.

Now all of a sudden, in the parking lot of Saint Ann's Hospital, Lyle noted a new kind of ambulance, a Ford Econoline Van with a specialized cab built onto its chassis, almost like a mini-mobile-motor home built right onto the Econoline. Lyle looked inside, seeing a kaleidoscopic array of equipment including oxygen ports built into the walls, intravenous solutions waiting to be hung, cardiac monitors, in those days weighing fifty pounds, and plastic airways that could be inserted right there in the Econoline

He saw one of the ambulance drivers in a blue uniform with the yellow letters EMT embroidered on her back. She was wearing a "tool" belt with pouches for her industrial-sized scissors, a stethoscope, a Swiss Army Knife, and a flashlight.

Lyle thought, "Surely she's still an unregulated Cadillac driver who might deliver a little first aid at best? After all, the ambulance driver only has to know a few pressure points, how to drive, get to the hospital, maybe take a short cut or two. But what's all this?"

Lyle quizzed the young woman in the blue uniform, Valerie Vincente, who said, "I'm an emergency medicine technician, no longer just an ambulance driver. The country's undergoing a radical departure from the old concepts of 'load and go' with acutely sick and injured patients. We're extending initial medical care from the confines of the hospital's brick and mortar into the homes, restaurants, and streets of the community. Why delay treatment until the patient arrives at the hospital? With intervention at the scene we can produce better patient outcomes, especially with heart attacks and trauma. Thousands of heart attacks strike every day in this country with most of the deaths occurring in the prehospital setting."

"But, wait a minute, just wait a minute, field intervention by former Cadillac ambulance drivers now chauffeuring sick people in mini-mobile-motor homes?" Lyle was baffled, literally groping for words. "How in God's name can they train ambulance drivers about the treatment of emergencies when they don't even train doctors about emergencies?"

After all, he had to learn about hot sugar burns on his own. None of this was making any sense to the ill-fitting Lyle on his way to the administrator's office to pick up his weekly kitchen scheduling check from the secretary.

Lyle had been kitchen scheduling for about three years when he decided to attend a meeting of an organization he'd recently heard about, the American Academy of Emergency Physicians. Surely they would know about the Econolines? If not, then he would tell them.

After he and Carolyn arrived in Atlanta, the site of the 1974 meeting, he first went to the exhibit area, looking at the latest medical and surgical textbooks, noting nothing new on hot sugar burns. Actually, there was no comprehensive textbook on the field of emergency medicine. This absence seemed to confirm Lyle's suspicion that this peripheral medical field was simply a temporary earn-as-you-learn physician experience, with a few oddball autodidacts here and there devoting their lives to the "accident room" response to a patient's sudden medical or surgical emergency.

Emergency medicine certainly didn't offer a conventional career destination to young physician graduates, and was indeed analogous to the early history of the state of Wyoming where Frederick Paxson once wrote, "Early Wyoming was a thoroughfare rather than a destination."

Lyle wandered about the exhibit hall, noting with apprehension a group of physicians who'd begun to do emergency medicine full-time instead of moving on to other fields. These physicians were a somewhat frightening lot in the early nineteen seventies, many with long hair and sandals, wearing beads and peace buttons, some cultivating the Charley Manson look, but ironically, when Lyle went to the lecture series, he found most of them to be quite learned in spite of their scraggly appearances.

The physicians who did emergency room work full-time were called the "scrubs," and more than a few of the "scrubs" had finished residency-training programs, some in surgery, some even in urology and ophthalmology, but mostly internal medicine or family practice, many looking for their niche. They were a slightly bizarre group of physicians from a bazaar of medical backgrounds now in search of a specialty, and these young, fledgling physicians were perfect pigeons for the new group of kitchen schedulers arising in different parts of the country.

After the lectures, Lyle hung around eavesdropping on various conversations. He became confused when he heard a group of physicians from the Rocky Mountain region and the Detroit area talking about raising emergency medicine to the full status of a medical specialty.

Lyle was astounded. "How can they make kitchen scheduling into a distinct medical specialty like surgery or pediatrics? That's the wackiest thing I've ever heard."

He became even more fearful of this emergency medicine crowd, but suddenly realized they weren't talking about the kitchen schedulers, but about the "scrubs," making the "scrubs" into a separate medical specialty, which made him wonder even more.

"How can they possibly train a physician so broadly in all fields of medicine? The cross-sectional information needed to treat the full spectrum of diverse emergencies is encyclopedic. It simply can't be mastered by one physician. This is as silly as former Cadillac chauffeurs called EMTs driving mobile-homes wearing tool belts." Lyle listened for a little while longer, but the conversation amongst these more academically oriented physicians "deteriorated" into toxicology and trauma, uninteresting topics to Norman so he slowly moved on.

He continued to note with much more interest a different kettle of fish, a whole gallery of kitchen schedulers from different parts of the country, and he began to feel an uneasy kinship with these M.D.'s who no longer practiced medicine, but were full-time kitchen schedulers for emergency rooms. He sat with his new lodge brothers, and while exchanging pleasantries Lyle ascertained most of the kitchen schedulers to be washouts of various residency programs, obvious second raters with a flimsy background of a one-year rotating internship under their belts. They seemed to be mostly disgruntled physicians who for nebulous reasons had gone to medical school, undistinguished men of fairly modest gifts who, in other times in other specialties, would have remained mere footnotes. Norman Lyle readily saw through their overdrawn claims to be "pioneers" of a new specialty called emergency medicine.

However, they did all go to a fine set of haberdashers, wearing suits instead of the sackcloth scrubs. In fact, they proudly distinguished themselves from the hippie "scrubs" by their "suits."

Lyle very happily buttoned the vest of his new pinstripe the former Carolyn Skanks had bought for him while witnessing the initial dichotomy of emergency medicine doctors between the kitchen scheduling "suits" and clinical "scrubs."

Lyle happened to notice a small group listening to a fellow named Goldman, who actually claimed to be "the founder of emergency medicine." Lyle was in awe listening to this clever, cliche-throwing poet laureate, but as he heard Goldman speak, he realized Goldman was nothing more than an overblown kitchen scheduler, an opportunist like himself filling in the blanks with "scrubs" in Upstate New York, and he was astonished Goldman was bragging about it.

Lyle almost busted out laughing when Goldman began speaking about the "perils of debt" for Lyle knew there was no investment, no need to bet the ranch. All one needed was a little seed money for a kitchen and a phone, and with a little hustle, one could kitchen schedule "scrubs" to fill in blanks. In reality, with a little beginner's luck and a pay phone, even a homeless person could kitchen schedule.

But Lyle felt the better part of his thinly-capitalized kitchen scheduling valor was stealth, and even though that ancestral feeling began to surface again, Lyle caught hold of himself. He'd been around the block a time or two, knowing this short-term aberration of gouging twenty-five per cent of the physician fee for kitchen scheduling wouldn't be tolerated but a few years by the general medical community, certainly never gaining mass acceptance by the membership of the American Medical Association.

Besides, Lyle was bemused, watching the founding of a medical specialty domineered by groups of individuals having no intention of ever practicing the specialty.

Lyle thought, "Surely a medical specialty can't be formed by a group of people having no intention of ever seeing a patient themselves, only kitchen scheduling 'scrubs' to fill in blanks, then calling the specialty emergency medicine? This lame-brain scheme to recognize a formal specialty can't possibly be successful, or for that matter, even legal."

He logically sided with those who felt a certain sense of urgency that the kitchen schedulers had to cash in within a short span of time because this blank canvas of opportunity wasn't going to last forever.

Listening to Goldman, Lyle sensed a certain insidiousness to these highly charged "suits," a salivation, something he couldn't call greed quite yet, but the lure of money was heavy in the air. Even more than that, he could feel the power, a slight sense, but ever so invigorating. Goldman blamed other physicians in other specialties for ignoring emergency medicine, and said that controls would have to be placed on the medical community. Goldman was laying the foundation to blame others for the wreckage, the wreckage they were all about to create in the systematic transfer of wealth and power out of the hands of those physicians who evaluated and treated patients into the hands of those who kitchen scheduled.

"This is just a ruse, a sham, a pyramid scheme," Lyle thought.

"A pyramid scheme," Norman suddenly clicked, and with a slight smile appearing on his face, he knew his new kitchen scheduling company would be called Pyramid, with its purpose to grow, simply to grow, forever broadening its base, constantly overreaching for kitchen scheduling blanks while bottom fishing for physicians to staff the "accident rooms" of New England, and now, the emergency rooms from sea to shining sea.

Lyle was in ecstasy with a broad smile on his face when suddenly Goldman pointed at him, thinking the grinning Lyle had a question, but Lyle thought Goldman wanted him to make a statement.

Lyle, in one of his rare moments of immaturity said, "It's kind of like the Roman Catholic Church, you just obtain a few pennies from all the people."

Goldman was obviously miffed, but there were a few chuckles in the audience, especially from a "scrub" named Kensington. That chance remark stuck to Lyle, and many years later he would grow to regret the offhanded remark very much.

Walking back to the hotel, Lyle didn't know how to view this seemingly benign occupation of the nation's emergency rooms by the kitchen schedulers, but he knew for the moment "someone had to do it." Without question, so long as he could stay out of clinical medicine and out of the sugar frosted flakes building, Norman Lyle had that willingness to serve.

The next day he moved about, listening carefully to talk of the recently enacted 1973 Emergency Medical Services Systems Act. The "suits" were buzzing about it, half of them fearful they might be found out, but the other half with a boomtown hysteria, speaking of the huge sums of money the United States Congress had appropriated. A half a billion dollars was the figure being bantered around with twenty million for New England alone. "That's a lot of Econolines," Lyle thought, watching the crime of the century unfold, ever so thrilled to be a part of it.

He also sensed the emerging philosophy of the kitchen schedulers. They had to be somewhat careful to dance on the edge of the rules, both written and unwritten. Lyle began to see the importance of this new organization with its original draftsmen in keeping information rationed and the rules unwritten. He noted the membership tables set up everywhere in the large hanger of the exhibit area extolling physicians to become members of the Academy. Lyle immediately saw how important it was for the "suits" to claim the mantle first, to become officialdom, be the spokespeople for emergency medicine before the "scrubs" or academics started their own organizations.

Norman said to Carolyn, "This could be an important career

move. I think we should personally pay the annual dues of the physicians who work for us to belong to the Academy."

"Yes, I agree. This so-called Academy will eventually want a cut of the action, and they'll certainly notice the sudden infusion of dues money from the new Pyramid," said Carolyn, "and I think a cozy association will encourage their cooperation in the future."

"It's so amazing Carolyn. Institutions are just the same everywhere, Boston politics, Tammany Hall, and now the party bosses of the American Academy of Emergency Physicians."

They chuckled, with Carolyn replying, "You know, this concept of an Academy does seem to elevate the pedestrianism of these 'founders' we've met."

They both laughed, with Norman saying, "With the initial language properly structured, we can get the upper hand for redistribution of the 'scrubs' income."

They then overheard one of the "suits" talking about a forty per cent kitchen scheduling fee.

"Forty per cent!" Lyle said. We can't get away with slicking forty per cent of the fees in Boston."

"Or can we?" the smiling Carolyn said, "now that we'll be on such chummy terms with the Academy, and two of their first insiders."

All the clever "fellows" of kitchen scheduling soon noted a staggering amount of wealth could be made by placing various and sundry physicians into empty slots, the blanks, in hospital emergency department schedules. After all, someone besides the nurses had to be there when the Econolines arrived driven by EMTs now carrying a living patient not quite ready for the black Cadillac.

And then to everyone's astonishment, out of nowhere, in the mid-seventies, a much more important and totally unexpected, utterly serendipitous boon to the economy of the "suits" occurred, improving their balance sheets more than they could have imagined. A highly-popular television series about EMTs and paramedics rose to the top of the Nielsen ratings, and hospital administrators all over the nation suddenly felt they "needed" a supply of doctors, preferably handsome well-spoken ones in their emergency rooms, but if necessary, hippie "scrubs" who knew what they were doing, or for that matter, anyone with an unrevoked license. The hospital administrators were perfect knockovers for the flimflam kitchen scheduling men eager for quick profits in this new specialty mushrooming overnight.

The kitchen schedulers were soon making so much money in their kitchens they would never pick up stethoscopes again. Several dropped out of lucrative ophthalmology and radiology practices just so they could make out schedules for emergency departments. Some maintained Ear, Nose and Throat practices while their wives made out the schedules on the side with their imprimatur on them. While it was true a physician could make a good living practicing medicine in an emergency room, the real bullion was in scheduling.

This sudden cornucopia of kitchen scheduling wealth created a population explosion of "suits," beginning to attract a large stream of rather slippery-eel "civilians" as well—insurance salesmen, used-car types, personal-injury lawyers, etc.—the quick studies seeing the thirty-three per cent profit margin in scheduling emergency rooms as irresistible temptation.

Kitchen scheduling soon became the fastest-growing specialty in medicine, a growth industry comparable to fast food or video rental stores, only the latter two had industry standards. The "suits" surprisingly noted there were no controls over where they placed the "generic" physicians, regardless of the physician's background or reputation, so they quickly suffered a precipitous decline in ethics and honesty. The kitchen schedulers, now formally freed from background checks by the Academy, placed dermatology residents in pediatric trauma hospitals, radiology residents in cardiac hospitals, but again, just kitchen scheduling any Tom, Dick, or Harry into any blank, anywhere, anytime.

Of course, Doctors Tom, Dick, and Harry had to have an active, unrevoked, state medical license. Otherwise it would be illegal and violate the law, not the rules. Actions that became known amongst the "suits" as "unethical" were actually only those activities the states' legislatures had expressly codified as illegal. After all, they had to have some written guidelines, and there were certainly no standards of integrity forthcoming from the thumbs up their asses at the now well-funded American Academy of Emergency Physicians.

There was no mechanism to limit the "suits' " vastly growing wealth—no laws, no codes, no rules, no regulations—nothing save their own sparse consciences. And although there were no systematic field studies verified with double-regression analysis, it was widely believed by everyone in the field in the nineteen seventies that the formation of the American Academy of Emergency Physicians, along with the premature introduction of full-time generic physician coverage, cost many an American life.

The "suits" also noticed they had huge amounts of time on their hands, many completing their schedules in the first week of the month. Because these washouts from rotating internships were never quite fitted to clinical medicine, this newly created leisure class began to do things other physicians didn't ordinarily do. With the constant infusion of money and limitless time, they took law and business classes learning all about corporations and partnerships. They were delighted to know they could be "CEO's" of their own clever little creations, enamored with the tax codes, studying right down to the commas and semicolons any sections affecting them. They learned how to bill insurance companies up the ying-yang, optimize if not slightly upcode, milk Medicare and, of course, fleece the "scrubs."

As for Jenny? Jenny's death was simply considered part of

the hidden cost of doing business, the business of emergency medicine, the real new specialty.

CHAPTER FOUR

ORIGIN OF A SPECIES

"To see patients without reading is like a ship without a rudder, to read and not see patients is like never having gone to sea."
—*Sir William Osler, M.D.*

Although Steinerman signed a two-year contract with Pyramid, Inc. to begin an odyssey working in different emergency rooms, he actually remained close to the greater Boston area for a number of reasons. He felt somewhat guilty about beginning the odyssey without Shelly, plus Mahoney, after finishing a one-year fellowship in pediatric emergency medicine, had moved back to the Boston area. Steinerman was beginning to realize what a recluse he'd become, consciously sensing his loneliness. It was very good to have Philip Mahoney around again. And there was another reason.

Steinerman wasn't quite prepared to be an emergency room doctor in a community hospital without any interns or residents. He felt mildly uneasy about being the only physician on the premises after midnight in a one-hundred-bed community hospital.

He hadn't realized how hard "easy" medicine was, having been used to dramatic illnesses and melodramatic treatments at the General. He'd treated rheumatic fever and poststreptococcal renal disease, the possible sequelae of an untreated strep throat, but he hadn't actually seen a patient with a simple strep throat in his eight years at Harvard. Although he knew all about Kaposi's Sarcoma, he'd never seen a case of impetigo. Conditions like tension headaches, coughs, constipation, ligament sprains, insect bites, minor fractures, anxiety, weakness, shoulder aches, and even uncomplicated vaginal discharges were all like new diseases to him.

When he went home at night, he read about them as intensely as he'd read about the three stages of Lyme disease or the nuances of congenital heart defects in the past. In his isolation he enjoyed the readings, slowly acquiring a comfortableness in the emergency room—that one-twentieth of an acre on the hospital's first floor where unscheduled, unrestricted, high-risk patients of all ages with all potential diseases presented themselves for immediate diagnosis and treatment.

Steinerman relieved Walsh one evening at the Brookline Methodist Hospital. They were both working in one of Lyle's many, many emergency room "management" contracts. Walsh was a well-known alcoholic who'd been thrown out of the internal medicine program for being swacked on the job too many times. He was a poor clinician and an asshole to boot. Walsh was in a rush, quickly telling Steinerman of the only patient he had left.

The patient was an eight-year-old boy named Ponce de Leon Rodriguez who'd presented with the chief complaint of shortness of breath. Walsh explained that "de Leon" was just waiting for a prescription, and could be released as soon as the medication arrived from the pharmacy. Steinerman said "o.k.," and was glad to see Walsh leave.

Steinerman's overall competence superseded his book learning and experience. His mind was intuitive, and his overall abilities had evolved to the point of reflexes, instinctual and glandular. He was a diagnostic animal, a jaguar or leopard always on the prowl for afflicted prey. Steinerman's father was proud of him, and for that matter, Maimonides himself would have been proud of Steinerman.

He noted de Leon's posture, a slight leaning forward, and he scented a color variation, an ever-so-slight bluish tint struggling to surface through de Leon's olive-brown skin. It went completely unnoticed by everyone, the nurses, his teachers, and even his family, but not to the big Cat.

Steinerman introduced himself to the family, letting them know he wanted to look the patient over one more time before they left. The Cat was circling. The nurses were pissed because de Leon was already "treated and streeted," but his family was grateful. One of the nurses had already written a note commenting on the delayed discharge on the "quality assurance" forms Pyramid, Inc. distributed monthly to the nursing staff.

But de Leon's family had instincts, too. They knew they were being cheated as they were the people who bought the five-hundred-dollar cars with the one-hundred-dollar monthly interest payments. They were used to getting the shit kicked out of them, and instinctively knew Walsh was a shit doctor giving them a bullshit prescription, and instinctively trusted the big Cat.

The cougar suddenly sprung as Steinerman listened to de Leon's chest. To his surprise the lungs were clear. He'd expected fluid in them. Approaching his stethoscope to de Leon's heart, he began to hear the rumble. The heart murmur was deafening, swish, swish, to and fro—so loud he wondered how de Leon slept at night. Surely Walsh had picked this up. He looked at Walsh's chart.

Color	WNL
Lungs	WNL
Heart	WNL

WNL is the commonly used medical abbreviation for **W**ithin **N**ormal **L**imits.

That shit Walsh hadn't even listened to de Leon's heart, prescribing Valium for the boy's anxiety. De Leon was short of breath because of anxiety? How fucking lazy can you get?

Steinerman called the nurses over, asking what WNL meant, and they all cried in unison, "Within normal limits," oblivious as usual to the obvious trap. Steinerman then had them listen one by one to de Leon's heart, and they were virtually in tears when Steinerman, the chief from the General, told them whenever they read **WNL** on Walsh's chart it meant **WE NEVER LOOKED.** That's right, **WNL** was no longer within normal limits, it was, *we never looked.*

De Leon was referred *that night* to a pediatric cardiac surgeon, Doctor Christine Kull. Kull told Steinerman that his note on the chart regarding the gallop, heart murmur, and final conclusion was the equivalent of the intracardiac catheter she'd placed, nicknaming him "the walking catheter."

Kull sewed the hole in de Leon's heart the next day, replaced one of his heart valves, and told Steinerman that de Leon would live longer than the both of them.

She wanted to know where Steinerman had done his electives in pediatric cardiology, and he laughingly replied, "Nowhere." In fact, he wasn't even a pediatrician. Doctor Christine Kull had suddenly met one of the large Cats in emergency medicine.

The rest of Steinerman's night was uneventful, a few sprained ankles and sore throats, and several girls from Radcliffe College with vaginal discharges.

Harvard students learn early on not to blemish their records, any records, and not to trust the confidentiality of any department—including the student health service. They are also aware of the large number of double-blind statistical studies going on in university hospitals, and do not trust the destination of the blood specimen leaving their arm. Everyone's well aware that being positive for the wrong substance or a particular virus isn't a smart thing to have recorded in the computer age. A spotless record can prove useful for snooping moms and dads, boyfriends, graduate schools, and those who might inquire about a top security clearance in the future.

So when signs of potential venereal disease show up, it's worth the trip and expense to go to a hospital several miles outside of Cambridge, leaving their own university medical records untarnished. A distant emergency room offers almost perfect anonymity for cash-paying students using a Jane Doe.

Of course, the Radcliffe women insisted on being creative, so when Steinerman saw patients' names on the chart like "Lady Di Smith" or "Dame Nancy Reagan," he knew he was in for a pelvic exam.

Apparently, one of the more prolific males had infected several of the more attractive coeds with trichomonas. The young women all complained of itchy, annoying, foul-smelling vaginal discharges. Trichomonas localizes to the vaginal vault and bladder neck, never spreading or invading the bloodstream. Therefore, the patients are never really "sick," and so from the physician's viewpoint, vaginitis is not an urgent problem. However, from the patient's perspective, it is a most uncomfortable and embarrassing disease.

The organism also lives asymptomatically in the prostate gland of the male never causing him any problems. It was rumored the male index case slept with a recently arrived Taiwanese graduate student, starting the "epidemic" and confirming a recent tradition in medicine of blaming orientals for contagious infectious disease pandemics such as Hong Kong, Shanghai A2, or the Bangkok flu.

Steinerman couldn't help but notice the copious, grayish, malodorous vaginal discharges during the pelvic exams, and after checking the vaginal pH, he proceeded to look at a drop of the discharge mixed with a drop of saline under the microscope. Looking at the "wet mount," he saw zillions of highly-motile, round, unicellular organisms whirling around bopping into one another, their flagellae whipping around too fast to be seen by the unaided eye, even under the microscope. The trichomonads seemed like dancing punk rockers having a grand old time playing roller derby, smacking into each other as hard as they could. Steinerman sent off cultures to check for other sexually transmitted diseases, not-uncommon co-infections with trichomoniasis.

He then gave the young duchesses their medication with a script for "Typhoid Trich" if they would care to give it to him. He warned the most common cause of recurrence is reinfection from re-exposure to the same partner, the infection many times "ping ponging" between cohorts if both are not treated simultaneously. The young ladies took the extra script, but insisted "Trich" was ancient history in their lives.

Steinerman believed Trichomonas infections had a mild, but representative diagnostic odor, not an undifferentiated, disagreeable genital smell, but a specific and characteristic odor, recognizable with "olfactory skills." Mahoney and several of the gynecologists disagreed with Steinerman, saying Trich infections didn't have any distinctive smell distinguishing them from other causes of vaginitis.

Steinerman saw over twenty patients on his twelve-hour night shift, most of them with minor complaints, staple illnesses. One twenty-two year old had pruitic (itchy), papules (bumps) on his penis, a dead giveaway for scabies infestation. PPP (**p**ruitic, **p**apules on the **p**enis) is not an infrequent abbreviation in medicine. Later that evening Steinerman saw an elderly man with long-standing Alzheimer's Disease from a nursing home who'd recently "stroked out." The patient had pinpoint pupils indicating a burst blood vessel in the area of the brain known as the pons, and fortunately for the individual and his family, this PPP (**p**inpoint **p**ontine **p**upils) indicated the patient did not have long to live. In the land before time before antibiotics, old men used to die of pneumonia long before they became senile and had to linger in the intensive care unit through the "one-hundred-thousand-dollar funeral." Sir William Osler referred to pneumonia as "the old man's friend."

A patient presented with sickle-cell crisis, along with two women with urinary tract infections, one depressed young woman insisting on a silver bullet chemical fix-it, one patient with a possible heart attack, two asthmatics, a young woman with diarrhea who'd recently traveled to Mexico, several kids from a karate class with nasty nasal and toe fractures (self-defense classes being known amongst emergency physicians as self-destruction classes), one child with croup, one adult with three days of intractable hiccups, two industrial accidents from the sugar frosted flakes factory, one malingerer in local police custody seeking a medical excuse to avoid a court appearance, and one schizophrenic who was less-than-faithfully taking his medications, not currently watching the same in-flight movie the rest of the world was.

The internist, orthopedist, cardiologist, psychiatrist, neurologist, pediatrician, and general practitioner Steinerman called to either come in and admit the patients, or to follow-up with them in their offices were cordial, competent, didn't ask about the insurance status of the patients, and ended the phone conversations with "Thank you for your help doctor." The only small physician problem Steinerman had was getting a patient transferred to the Veteran's Hospital at two a.m.

At the " V.A." Hospital, there existed the finest "goalies" in all of medicine, physicians who came to work, warmed up a bit, took a shower, put on mask and gloves, and sharpened their skates knowing that no Gordie Howes would slip an emphysematous, retired buck sergeant or cirrhotic naval boozer into their net. They were doctors who had over seventy file cabinets full of the proper responses to refuse any patient from any of the uniformed services with any disease. But Steinerman had the Stanley Cup when it came to the "V.A." His patient, a seventy-two year old war hero, was clearly heard shouting in the background, "I've had more pussy than any other vet. I've fucked everything from a pygmy to an Eskimo, but not a one of them ever measured up to my mother." Even with that introduction, Steinerman, to the cheers of the nurses, slapped that patient into the net of the Roxbury V.A.

The next day Steinerman called Mahoney for lunch, but Mahoney had to testify on a rape case. Steinerman said he would go with him since he'd never been to court.

The case involved a twenty-three year old laboratory technician who'd been raped and beaten on her way home from work six months ago.

Mahoney was the first to see her in the emergency room. The staff gynecologist was tied up in the operating room, and Mahoney proceeded with the formal rape exam according to the guidelines Delorenzo had set up in Hershey, Pennsylvania. Joe Delorenzo established the sexual-assault examination procedures while in his emergency medicine residency program, and it was becoming the nationwide standard of care for the medical rape exam. Its methodology and chain of evidence protocol were also becoming legally acceptable for conviction in all fifty states.

The young woman had surprisingly little vaginal bleeding secondary to a broken Coke bottle placed into her vagina after the assault. Mahoney had taken a swab of the vaginal drippings, looking at it himself under the microscope. He readily saw millions of sperm swimming in Brownian motion, hundreds of millions of ugly, deranged, psychopathic sperm, aimlessly swimming against the tide, probably pathogenic sperm full of God knows what—gonorrhea, syphilis, AIDS, and the awful potential of pregnancy. Mahoney stabilized the young woman, assisting as the victim was taken to the operating room because there was too much reactive spasm in the vaginal walls to remove the glass without general anesthesia. They needed perfect relaxation of the vaginal musculature which came only under "general."

The gynecologist in the operating room had just finished his last case of the day, but Mahoney told him not to leave—they were on their way up. She had a full stomach but there was no way around surgery now, regardless of the risk she might vomit and aspirate the vomitus into her lungs. Fortunately, they did take her into the operating theater that night because one of the longer pieces of glass had penetrated the vaginal wall perforating the peritoneum. She required exploration of the belly where they found a punctured ovary and several bleeding vessels, along with a tear in the wall of the colon with extravasation of fecal contents throughout the peritoneal cavity. She did well in surgery, but required a colostomy, having to spend six months with a bag of shit zippered to her belly, and was now well enough to testify.

Steinerman watched the defendant's attorney badger Mahoney relentlessly, obviously angered by Mahoney's quickness and jury appeal. The defendant's attorney knew he had to discredit Mahoney.

"Dr. Mahoney, you're not a gynecologist, are you?"

"No sir."

"Dr. Mahoney, you said you looked at the vaginal secretions and saw sperm, right?"

"Yes sir."

"Dr. Mahoney, how long is the flagella on a sperm?"

"I don't know, sir"

"You don't know, but then again you're not a specialist in gynecology. And there's a lot about gynecology you're not expected to know. How many microns long, then, is the flagella on a trichomonad?"

"I don't know."

"You don't know. But there you are, wanting to send a man to jail for many years, possibly for life, and you can't tell the difference in the lengths of the flagellae between two motile, very similar appearing cells under the microscope. That really sounds like beyond a reasonable doubt to me?"

"Yes, but you see..."

"That's all, your honor, no more questions. The witness may step down. He's already told us enough of what he's not sure of."

"Your honor, if I may."

The heavy set, mustached, bald headed judge, David Jones, who knew Mahoney from previous trials, leaned back in his large leather chair, and slowly mumbled, "Go ahead, Dr. Mahoney."

Steinerman watched the other large Cat circle. Mahoney continued, looking straight into the eyes of every member of the jury.

"If there were a Chinese girl and a Caucasian girl walking down the street together, both with black shiny hair, and if they both wore an identical set of clothing from head to toe, and were exactly the same height, and were walking right next to each other, one might say they looked very much alike. But if you asked me which one was the Chinese girl and which one the Caucasian girl, I think you could believe me if I said I could distinguish them beyond a reasonable doubt. That's exactly how sure I am there were millions of sperm in that vaginal sample and not trichomonads."

A devastating silence ensued as Mahoney quietly stepped down. The rest of the trial was *fait accompli* after Mahoney had sprung on them.

Steinerman felt a growing respect for these residency-trained emergency physicians. A new breed of Cats was on the horizon, but someone needed to eliminate the poachers before these agile jaguars were here today and gone tomorrow, extinct, gone to other specialties, specialties without pledge drivers, "suits," or thumbs up their asses.

CHAPTER FIVE

CRIPS AND BLOODS

> "These fellas did what Senators have been doing for a long time. There's nothing illegal about it. It's just wrong."
> —*Senator William Proxmire*

Norman Lyle, just returned from his tenth consecutive pilgrimage to the annual conclave of the American Academy of Emergency Physicians, had undergone his own evolution through the years.

He and Carolyn, along with the other kitchen schedulers, had never liked their name, so they and the Academy changed it to "managers." The kitchen schedulers then begat more money to "manage," since something must have changed other than their names. The "scrubs," still seeing the patients, hadn't changed their names, so they were kept at scale.

Lyle had also learned the only way to obtain more lucrative emergency room contracts to kitchen schedule was to secure the hospital administrator's vote of confidence in any way possible. Although the medical staff would rubber stamp an individual physician in order to grant him or her hospital privileges, the actual hiring and firing of the "management" group was done solely through the hospital administrator, and this was the only specialty in medicine where the administrator held such power over the doctors.

Hospital administrators themselves were a heterogeneous lot of Cats and kittens in the nineteen seventies and eighties, coming from many walks of life, and, like many of the emergency medicine physicians, had no formal training for the job. They pretty much **o**n-**t**he-**j**ob-trained themselves for their positions, thus earning the nickname **O-J-T**-ers. There were a few possessing public health degrees in hospital administration, but most came up through the ranks of the hospital's subculture or, for that matter, many came out of nowhere—former strategic air command pilots, bank loan officers, salesmen of medical equipment, and Lutheran ministers. Many were quite good, running pretty tight ships, and more than a few had a gift for fundraising.

But many were somewhat buffoonish and sometimes, many times in fact, one had to think there were bands of number-crunching accountants and assorted pointy-heads in the basements of many, many hospitals keeping the ships afloat.

One thing was clear though, it was the hospital administrator who singlehandedly decided which group of kitchen schedulers would "manage" his or her emergency department—not the physician staff, not the board of directors, not a mechanism in the hospital bylaws, but it was solely the administrator who determined on which side the "suits'" bread was buttered.

The late 1970's and early eighties represented years of unprecedented violence for emergency medicine as the mad dash to become wealthy kitchen schedulers had saturated the scheduling market, but, up until this point, the "suits" played by the Marquess of Queensbury's rules.

The "suits'" problems all began within a three hundred square mile area of the country whose name will be withheld to protect the innocent, just in case there are any. The anonymous midwestern "region" (surrounded by an area where a very famous auto race is held every year) contained twenty hospitals, all with active emergency rooms. The "region" had a large city with a medical school assuring a supply of residents in various specialty training programs, a clearinghouse of generic physicians.

Two groups, the "suits" and the "rival suits," gerrymandered the contracts with the twenty hospitals in "the region" evenly, and each of the non-physician M.D. "suits" made over a million dollars a year, and, of course, never saw patients, only went to law, tax, and "management" seminars. But for the "suits," it wasn't enough, because market saturation stagnation had set in.

One day, one of the "suits" was driving by one of the "rival suits'" contract hospitals when a particularly mischievous thought entered his mind. He stopped and demanded to see the hospital administrator. As it turned out, the O-J-T-er had gone to the same college as the "suit," and the "suit" took him out for lunch at a fancy country club. The "suit" told the O-J-T-er how he was being cheated by the "rival suit." He said he could provide much better doctors, even though everyone used the same generics, more than a few Monks, and an occasional Mahoney or Steinerman. Playing through the eighteen holes that afternoon, the "suit" told the administrator how the other kitchen schedulers were one dimensional, and he could provide many more "services" to the hospital, the "services" very sketchily described. The O-J-T-er promptly dropped the "rival suits'" emergency medicine "management" contract changing the scoreboard to 11-9 in favor of the "suits."

The "rival suits" were shocked, experiencing a touch of *the horror* themselves at this dispicable act on the part of the "suits." They belabored the ethics of the atrocity, calling upon the works of Kant, Hegel, the constitution, eastern religions, and Galen. Although the terminology had not yet evolved, it was clear to the "rival suits," they were the first victims of the most treacherous and cowardly of acts as "the region" recorded its first drive by shooting, emergency medicine style. The "rival suits" stayed in a state of confusion and disarray until one of their "consultants" suggested they hire a marketing expert.

"We need a marketing expert to outmaneuver these 'suits,' " said a recently hired MBA of the "rival suits' " organization. And thus the marketing of the emergency medicine contract "management" groups became the latest development in the ever more complicated and overcrowded world of kitchen scheduling which was now called "management." They had to market the same generic physicians and Monks to the same hospitals for the same amount of money; but the skimmed money, the scheduling commission, the Norman Lyle twenty-five to thirty-three per cent of gross, was paid to a different set of "suits," a different set of "managers," a different set of kitchen schedulers all armed with the same Rolodexes. The "suits" were hit with the rude awakening that the days of easy growth were over. The frontier was closing for the "pioneers" when marketing hit, and a good up-to-date Rolodex wasn't enough. The "suits" and "rival suits" needed new client lists with more blanks to fill in to keep up the days of heady growth.

And so a highly competitive turf battle begat the crips and the bloods of emergency medicine with the rival gangs trying to emerge as dominant players, dominant kitchen schedulers of the same generics. Pretty soon numerous splinter groups arose to challenge the crips and the bloods. Turf battles began to rage, and drive by shootings in emergency medicine became a daily occurrence.

A particularly sly emergency medicine street gang from the upper-midwestern peninsula "region" were a bunch of soft, roly-poly "suits" known for their craftiness, and rather pejoratively referred to by the bloods as "The Croissants." The "Bunkies" flourished throughout the whole North Texas "region," and a vicious group arose in the southwest called the "G. LiDDys." It was rumored the "G. LiDDys" once bit the head off a rabid bat, spitting it at the O-J-T-er, horrifying him into awarding them the "management" contract, also causing the regional poison control center to recommend a live rabies vaccine for the O-J-T-er. But for practical purposes, one can simply refer to the various emergency medicine "management" groups as the crips and the bloods.

Good golfing weather sent up small craft warnings to the "management" groups, and during one fine week in May, there were six "fatal" drive by shootings in "the region," as the "management" contracts kept changing hands. The emergency medicine crips and bloods became fiercely territorial and expansionistic, and in one ten-mile radius, there were two incidents within a span of thirty minutes. Actually, no one really noticed since the generics, the actual working doctors attired in "scrubs," never seemed to change, regardless of which crip or blood held the "management" contract.

The only notable difference in the region was the size of the hospital administrators, the O-J-T-ers. With so many rich luncheons to go to with the marketers, replete with caviar and Dom Perignon, the O-J-T-ers were beginning to look a little porked out from their afternoon cholesterol stress tests. Their country club extravagance, a true occupational hazard, began to take its toll, and at one luncheon an O-J-T-er suddenly collapsed.

The "suits" watched in horror not knowing what to do. To Heimlich or not to Heimlich, that was the question! None of them had taken any CPR (CardioPulmonary Resuscitation) courses, the raison d'etre of emergency medicine, and they vainly tried to apply the tax law to a dying man. They watched in horror as he writhed in convulsions, suddenly turning sky-blue. He bled from the edges of his tongue, a truly disgusting sight, and one of the marketers developed such an aversion to Beluga and Perignon he had to seek other employment. They waited for the ambulance, but by the time the Econoline arrived, the well-fed, coronary occluded O-J-T-er was already in rigor mortis. It just seemed like everyone was getting a bit of *the horror* these days.

The marketers became dismayed by the fact they were always offering the same generics to the same hospitals, and wanted to know if a subset of physicians working in the emergency rooms might become "their" doctors. Somehow, the highly competitive crips and bloods had to set themselves apart from the other major gangs in the booming kitchen scheduling marketplace. It would be quite a coup to have a Steinerman or Mahoney bound exclusively to work in "their hospital" which seemed an impossible feat at the time. The "suits" pondered the problem like Talmudic scholars, and the answer sprung from a most unlikely source, one of the attorneys in their growing legal departments, a specialist in contract law.

He suggested making the "scrubs" sign what was called a noncompete clause, forbidding them to work for the "rival suits." It initially seemed like a ludicrous concept that couldn't work in American medicine, and Lyle himself was against it at first. He couldn't see the upside potential of the gangs each having several well-hooked fish. He knew first hand the problems of the Rolodex, feeling revolving-door physicians for everyone made good business sense.

But after some study, the "suits" came up with a noncompete clause that was pure genius. In order to work, the "scrubs" had to sign an agreement not to work for any "rival suit" in the same hospital for a period of two years. This shotgun marriage ensured that if a "rival suit" had a successful drive by, the "scrub" working there wouldn't be allowed to work again in the same hospital for two years. In case any of the "suits" were victims of a drive by, they could forbid the generics from jumping ship and working there for anyone else. The noncompete clause, a simple spoil-sport measure, gridlocked physicians into and out of different hospitals. The "rival suits" would then have to work harder with the Rolodexes, spending more advertising money, taking more out of the physicians' fees because a new set of generic physicians would have to be found, and there was a limited pool of generics.

So with the Academy's backing, the "suits" sent out a double-barrel warning to the "scrubs" of the new gunboat diplomacy in effect in emergency medicine. The "scrubs" knew the crips and the bloods had quite a nasty streak, with a growing legal phalanx to sledgehammer them with the newest aspect of the delivery of emergency care to the American public and their children.

And thus the Rolodex containing the names of physicians with active, unrevoked, state medical licenses who were willing to work in an emergency room, to cover, to fill in a blank, became even more complicated. A current Rolodex now had to include the hospitals, what kind, where, and when the "scrubs" had signed a noncompete clause. The Rolodex became the most important part of "management" in the information age.

Now known in emergency medicine circles as the "recruitment department," the Rolodex was an important piece of "proprietary information," a trade secret not to be shared as the scheduling kitchens fortified themselves like Fort Ticonderoga. The Rolodex contained the names of residents and, unknown to the general medical world until this time, a reservoir of knockabout misfits with M.D. degrees who were more than willing to fill in a blank.

The crips and the bloods made the "scrubs" sign exclusivity contracts—paperwork barriers treating the "scrubs" like the Jackson Five, complicated contracts, sometimes twenty pages long with elaborate restrictions on working in a client hospital for a rival blood. The noncompete clause consisted of a hundred words hidden in the "whereases" section in the fine print of the single-spaced, Byzantine agreements, not that the medical or surgical residents read anything they signed anyway.

These exclusivity contracts, a form of wearing "colors," actually began to differentiate the "scrubs," and free agents became a dying breed further trivializing the physician's role in emergency medicine. The Mahoneys and Steinermans of the world were now quarantined from working in certain emergency rooms because of contracts they'd signed as residents, and would be rubber hosed into submission if they objected. The ball and chain noncompete clauses paved the way for the "suits" to cut the heart out of the new specialty. This little piece of chicanery, demanding physician fealty in writing to create an ineligibility status of fine physicians to work in certain community hospitals, was a brilliant marketing strategy, given the whole-hearted tacit approval of the thumbs up their asses at the American Academy of Emergency Physicians. Tacit approval, and that in itself spoke volumes about the Academy.

On the other hand, many of the founding members of the American Academy were the first leaders of the crips and the bloods. To these original shills of emergency medicine, the deep complicity in the duplicity, wheeler dealerism, and fiscal coups of any kind were simply good medicine, good emergency medicine.

The G. LiDDys never did join the Academy.

CHAPTER SIX

THE ANDERSON SYNDROME

"The only missing clotting factor is silk."
—*Donald Trunkey, M.D.*

It was Valerie Longo who first introduced Norman Lyle to Dan Anderson. Valerie was a well-known, competent, critical-care nurse at the General, rotating through the intensive and coronary care units and the emergency room. She worked for several hospitals on call, and although she was a little bossy, the critical-care units in Boston liked having Valerie for an evening shift; and when they had her, they almost always asked if she could work a double. She was energetic, a very meticulous organizer, and during her break time no less, she would rummage through the bedlam of the supply room, placing order in the linen and medicine closets.

One night an intravenous solution was ordered by the cardiologist to correct a patient's irregular heart rhythm, but a premixed, anti-asthma medication was hung by mistake, speeding up the patient's heart rate, increasing rather than decreasing the heart's irritability and irregularity. Since the medication was ordered at a very slow, electronically-controlled intravenous drip, the error wasn't noticed until the one liter bag completely ran out two days later.

Valerie, then, singlehandedly decided to place all premixed

intravenous solutions in different cabinets rather than all next to one other to decrease the risk of such understandable errors in the future. She did this in several different departments in several different hospitals with the utmost of efficiency, bypassing all committees and bureaucracies, her attitude simply being, "If they don't like it, they can change it back."

Although she exhibited fine clinical skills, everyone knew Valerie was destined for administration. She took night courses toward a masters degree of science in nursing, a common educational mistake of many sincere young men and women wishing to get ahead. She took hour after semester hour of coursework in communication skills, shocking everyone one day by announcing she was an expert in "effectively communicating" with abusive, hostile, even violent patients, requesting to be called for her professional consultation if any such human beings happened to stroll into the emergency room.

It took about an hour and a half for the next noble savage with an attitude to arrive at the General, and Valerie Longo R.N., M.S.N., was promptly called.

Steinerman was a resident at the time, and watched Valerie take charge, barking out orders to the other nurses, demanding a cup of coffee and a doughnut, and preparing to offer the provisions to the elderly woman who was kicking and screaming obscenities, and refusing to get out of her automobile at the front door of the emergency department.

Going out the door, the lion tamer explained to the nurses that offering coffee and doughnuts to a hostile patient often breaks the ice, allowing them "to begin a dialogue of effective communication." She said the most important reason for conflict of any kind was the breakdown of "effective communication," and she would elaborate later on the principles of crisis intervention, and in the future they would all role play as she had done many times in graduate school. Everyone was very impressed. Valerie was gone about ten minutes, and the ruckus outside seemed to have subsided when the loud crack was heard. It sounded more like a gunshot or an Achilles' tendon snapping in half than a slap in the face, but a faceslap it was, and the raging Valerie stormed through the front door with hemifacial swelling and marked redness, along with several small hot coffee burns on her wrists.

"That fucking bitch can go straight to jail," the communicator screamed, and when Steinerman asked to look at the burns on her wrist, Valerie refused. She was never called again for abusive patients although she continued to teach a very popular graduate school course on dealing with violent behavior.

Soon after the incident, Valerie went to work for Norman Lyle and Pyramid, Inc., Valerie becoming a gal-Friday type who did meticulous organizing for the meetings of Lyle and his henchmen with hospital administrators. She liked her job immensely, and credited her communication skills and her ability to "perceive the needs" of others as one of the main reasons for Pyramid's success in obtaining "management" contracts.

Valerie also fell secretly in love with Norman, an unrequited love because Lyle, who never stepped out, remained forever bonded to the former Carolyn Skanks via the kitchen table, but it was nevertheless an exciting and ongoing fantasy for Valerie. She liked being physically around Lyle, and loved to hear him speak, or softly sing vespers or evensong Gregorian chants in his office with his rich baritone. It was sometimes embarrassing for her to be around Lyle because her vaginal mucosal cells would hypersecrete in his presence, and sometimes she feared there was an odor in the air coming from her vaginal vault.

After Valerie introduced Lyle to Dan Anderson, he and Anderson had a short-term business relationship. Anderson knew of Valerie from his nurses, and when she called to request a meeting with him concerning a contract to provide emergency medicine doctors to his hospital, Dan Anderson was actually quite pleased. He had no idea at the time this would lead to a disease being named after him.

Dan Anderson was a very competent administrator at St. Joseph's Hospital in Boston. He had a somewhat blunt frontier style, taking little to no shit from the staff doctors. They liked him though, and St. Joseph's was one of the first to buy the CAT scanners, use ultrasound extensively, and integrate its emergency department with the newly implemented prehospital care system of paramedics. He upgraded the ICU (intensive care unit) and developed a separate neurological ICU for head-injured patients. He helped take obstetrics out of the dark ages, removing the medieval torture chambers otherwise known as delivery rooms, replacing them with a more civilized state of the art "birthing center." Anderson's progressive policies also demanded a high quality physician in the emergency department, one of the central hubs of a very busy hospital like St. Joseph's. The "declaration" of many a head-injured child was determined by the first few minutes of make or break care, and in fact, many critical patients had their fate determined within that first "Golden Hour" in the emergency department. There wasn't much point in having a sophisticated ICU if the patient's care was mucked up in the emergency room.

Anderson never understood why the emergency room was such an orphan in medicine. He could see the vast opportunity it held to give patients appropriate initial care, initial care so crucial to a successful outcome, but he saw the emergency physician was clearly the weakest link in the evolving emergency-medical-care system. The paramedics gave advanced care in the Econolines before even reaching the hospital, but most of the time, the "on call" physician was unsuitable.

On Wednesdays, the pediatrician was on E.R. call, which was fine except that one couldn't guarantee only children would get sick on Wednesday. The surgeon was on call Tuesdays, the orthopods on Mondays, and so on. The day to day operations of the emergency room didn't run quite as smoothly as the television show's rendition, and the chaos could best be described as a controlled crash with the nurses handling most of the problems, and the doctors—well, the doctors had to live and refer to one another, so they found it best not to complain about each other in front of outside groups if things went awry.

The staff doctors did, however, express their desire to be relieved of all emergency-room coverage forever if this was at all possible without fully abrogating their own responsibilities.

Therefore, after meeting with Valerie and Lyle, Anderson hired Pyramid, Inc. to "manage" his emergency department.

St. Joe's got Doctor Bing for a few seamless weeks, but then was saddled with both Monk and Walsh. Monk was buying a new house and filled many blanks, while Walsh—well, who really knows why, but he filled in most of the other blanks. After three months of this gruesome twosome, the staff doctors were up in arms, going directly to the hospital's board of directors, demanding an end to the carnage taking place under Pyramid's "management."

It should be emphasized they didn't actually want to return to emergency-room coverage themselves, but they knew the situation was infinitely worse under Pyramid, Inc. than it had been. Anderson told them he was doing his best with the hospital attorneys to bust the one-year contract with Pyramid, Inc., but they would be running into all kinds of lengthy legal problems.

Anderson also told them, "The few good residents who work here on weekends can't be hired back if we change groups."

"Why the hell can't they?" several staff physicians asked.

"Because they've signed a noncompete clause with Pyramid."

"What the hell is a noncompete clause?" the staff physicians demanded to know, but Anderson was incapable of explaining exactly what this new phenomenon in medicine was. Besides, the staff physicians would have been wholly incapable of understanding it, even had Anderson known, and everyone was certainly incapable of believing it.

"We'll also be hit with multiple lawsuits if we try to throw Walsh or Monk off the staff or if we renege on the rest of our contract with Pyramid."

The pediatricians, looking a little frayed around the edges from so many belligerent calls from unhappy parents, demanded to know what happened to Bing. Did Anderson, with that gruff manner of his, drive Bing out?

Anderson simply didn't have any answers, and Pyramid, Inc. wasn't about to tell him Bing was stretched to the bone with all the new contracts they'd obtained from their recent aggressive marketing campaign and the popularity of the new television series. Anderson was told to do something and do it now.

Anderson went through his file cabinet. He had over a hundred, glossy advertisements from different contract groups and individuals throughout the country offering to serve the "emergency needs of *your* hospital." He'd recently experienced a tidal wave of these slickly-written advertisements printed on fine, glossy, acid-free, very expensive stationary. He also noted the return addresses were always from areas like One Successful Road or Executiveland, U.S.A., a suburb of Happy Gardens in Prosperity County.

These overpackaged junk mailings were known in the emergency medicine trade as "glossies." The glossies, Hallmark-like greeting cards, were mellifluously-written, artfully-contrived, jargon-filled brochures, pictured with doctors in white coats wearing representative ties photographed in atmospheric settings.

"Who *are* these people?" Anderson wondered. He surprised himself since he'd never thought about it before. "Who the hell are these people and their organizations?" Anderson became concerned he was becoming part of a national bad joke. He'd never received glossies with 800 phone numbers advertising large orthopedic groups ready to supply his bone needs or neurosurgical companies with a ready supply of specialists to staff his brain needs. All the hype-filled glossies read the same:

> *...a board-prepared emergency medicine specialist who will live in your community. Our physicians take an active role on hospital committees, and heavily involve themselves in the community. They are trained personable professionals who want to be active participants in the development of your hospital emergency medical-care system. They have the extensive resources of our dedicated management group at their fingertips. A close ongoing relationship is an integral part of our service to you.*

It seemed that every other word and each little ditty had a circled, superscripted symbol next to it; every cute little expression for quality was registered®, serviced marked℠ copyrighted© or trademarked™ and the rhetoric in all the glossies went on and on, always ending with that magic word, the buzzword of the eighties, "Yes, Mr. Hospital Administrator, the bottom line of our group is **QUALITY**."

Anderson readily saw the bottom line of their group was clearly nothing other than the bottom line, and although he knew he was being conned with semi-truths and not-so-white lies, he needed to do something quickly. He called Goldman who came over himself the next day. Goldman intently listened to Anderson, empathizing with his woes, and sometimes expressing disbelief that such a thing could be happening.

Goldman took the contract, reassuring Anderson that Monk and Walsh would be traded for future draft picks, and the following week all ties were broken with Pyramid, Inc. Things went very well while Goldman's ace in the hole, initial start-up doctors charmed the entire staff during the first month's maiden voyage. But Goldman had growing pains, too, and pretty soon the initial boys in the white coats were slowly removed and placed in other new contract hospitals while the banana boat full of Goldman's second string mediocrities slowly inched its way up the Charles River, awaiting the word to dock and unload.

Six months to the day after throwing Pyramid, Inc. out, Anderson was horrified to learn Monk was back in the St. Joseph's Hospital emergency room working for Goldman's group, and Walsh was soon to follow. Goldman's Rolodex had simply run out of names.

Anderson called Goldman who bullshitted for a while saying Monk had improved greatly after attending the cardiogram seminars, and Walsh had stopped drinking. Goldman finally relented, saying they would be replaced, but Goldman had overcommitted his resources, and had run out of docs with unrevoked licenses.

It was mid-July, the most difficult of the fill-in-the-blank months, July being the traditional New Year for all of medicine. If anyone was moving they did it in July. His pledge drivers were on overtime running through their Rolodexes of possible "scrubs." He juggled as much as he could, but the two repackaged, rehabilitated retreads on the comeback trail would have to remain scheduled for at least a few shifts per month until September, until Goldman's outreach programs could hornswoggle a few new resident "scrubs."

Anderson was called before the hospital's medical staff and board of directors. He told them straightforwardly what had happened, but the "audience" knew that no situation like this existed in any other field of medicine, and weren't about to believe it existed in emergency medicine. They felt Anderson might be losing his edge because the story was simply too unbelievable. Anderson had spent so much time getting the emergency room fiasco squared away he wasn't as visible as he used to be in other areas of the hospital, and his absence was noted by many. The next day the chairman of the board of directors of St. Joseph's Hospital called Anderson in—he was fired.

This musical-chair policy of emergency medicine "management" groups became very well known in hospital circles. Administrators learned to be very careful before firing and replacing groups, and ending up with exactly the same doctors after the honeymoon and noncompete periods were over. O-J-T-ers knew, come hell or high water, they had to keep the "management" group or look like a fool to the hospital's board of directors. It was not wise for an administrator to admit openly to the board of directors that he or she had made an error in judgment, that they'd been bamboozled. The O-J-T-ers were just practicing a little preventive medicine, taking the prophylaxis against these potential pathogens, careful not to acquire the Anderson Syndrome themselves.

The "suits" quickly learned about the Anderson Syndrome, and knew the initial marketing and staged presentation of their "management" groups was everything. Whatever happened afterwards was secondary, and no matter how shady or outright crooked the emergency medicine "management" group turned out to be, no matter how falsely they represented themselves or the quality of their merchandise, the group would remain the incumbents for some face-saving time. The Anderson Syndrome was to play a pivotal role in the unraveling saga of the growth of organized emergency medicine. After the emergency medicine "management" contract was signed with the hospital, the crips and the bloods knew they had a stranglehold on the administrator, and devoted their resources to procuring new contracts by bushwhacking other unsuspecting O-J-T-ers.

After Monk was thrown out of St. Joseph's Hospital for the second time that year, he was quickly picked up by Pyramid's resettlement program, and moved back again to Dupage. Norman Lyle had expanded his operations into Southern Indiana early in 1981, and although he didn't like traveling to the Midwest, the small-town community hospitals in the corn and wheat field Serengetis made it an extremely lucrative region. After only two weeks back at the Dupage Community Hospital, Monk crash landed again.

Monk came in early one Monday morning to attend Morbidity and Mortality conference. He'd been "invited to attend" by the Chief of Surgery, Dr. Riley. The Chiefs of Surgery and Pathology hand-picked the cases for review.

Morbidity and Mortality conference, also known as **M** and **M**, consisted of a thorough review of a particular case, usually one that had been botched, and was attended by the medical students, nurses, and the entire variety of medical specialists. Nowhere were pathologists, surgeons, internists, pediatricians, emergency physicians, radiologists, and even public health specialists gathered together but at **M** and **M**. They were there to release their rancor, not their angst, but their invective as they challenged other physicians to defend their actions; **M** and **M** conferences were a great time to gang up on the primary "actor" who fucked up.

M and **M** days were also nicknamed **D** and **D**, **D**eath and **D**oughnuts, because the conferences were held early in the morning, the patients had invariably met a sticky end, and a most impressive variety of doughnuts was served. Pathology and surgery, much more than internal medicine, knew how to throw a conference. The primary actor sat on a stool on an empty stage, listening as the case was presented the way it had unfolded. Riley called for silence, announced today's case, and Monk prepared.

The case involved Mary G., a thirty-four year old housewife in good medical health. She was an unrestrained driver hit head on by a drunk driver at three o'clock in the afternoon. She presented with severe, left-upper-quadrant abdominal pain—the location of the spleen.

The spleen is the most vulnerable organ in blunt abdominal trauma, pediatric or adult. It's a solid organ laced with innumerable blood vessels, and bleeds profusely when ruptured. For a ruptured spleen, early recognition is necessary, and surgery in adults is almost invariably required.

Mary G.'s spleen was actually more shattered than ruptured, making its early removal with prompt control of bleeding mandatory for patient salvage. Her blood pressure was somewhat low and pulse rapid, both early warning signs of impending shock, but she was conscious, alert, and oriented. Monk gave her narcotics for her increasingly severe abdominal pain. Taking away the pain also removed her only symptom, the pain itself, leaving her to hemorrhage *painlessly*. Monk was, as they say, driving too slow for road conditions. While in x-ray for a useless, plain x-ray film of her abdomen, Mary G. "crashed." Monk raced to the radiology suite, immediately putting Mary G. on an intravenous "pressor" medication drip to increase her blood pressure, but actually the blood-pressure medicine squeezed her blood vessels down accelerating her bleeding. The medicine constricted her blood vessel walls forcing reluctant red blood cells out of their natural piping into the rising lake of blood sitting in her belly. Her abdomen became visibly distended.

What she needed was blood, the rapid administration of blood and many pints of it, blood and emergency surgery. She needed a surgeon to find the spleen, remove it, and tie off the lacerated blood vessels with silk sutures to stop her continued bleeding. She got none, only morphine and blood vessel constricting medications. Monk failed to notice Mary G wasn't breathing either. Monk had struck again. Mary G. couldn't be resuscitated, and was pronounced dead in the radiology department.

The audience groaned, staring in disbelief at this incompetent doctor sitting on the stool, out there in that big emergency room, a little money-making machine for Lyle, filling in the blanks for Pyramid, Inc.

Riley: "Let's now ask the pathologist to review the autopsy."

Paul Adkins said the cause of death was fairly easy to determine. Three liters or sixty per cent of the patient's blood volume was in her belly. The spleen was fragmented. Otherwise, there was minimal damage to other organs with some minor bruising of the bowel. There were petechiae and ecchymoses throughout both lung fields indicating pulmonary contusions or bruised, black and blue lungs, but this contributed little to the cause of death. Also, on routine toxicology studies, a dangerously elevated blood level of morphine was found. In other words, Mary G. was a completely preventable death of the worst kind. She came in alive and conscious, a death known in emergency medicine circles as the "talk and die" patient. (Jenny's death was known as the "go home and die" patient.)

CAUSE OF DEATH

1. Exsaunginating hemorrhage secondary to a ruptured spleen.
2. Respiratory depression due to excessive morphine administration.

Adkins added no one recorded on the chart the infusion of the vasoconstrictor. It didn't make much difference other than these compound errors were making Monk the eighth medical wonder of the world.

Riley: "Are we to understand, Dr. Monk, that not only did you not properly respond to the respiratory arrest of Mary G., but that you were also the one who gave her the excessive morphine in the first place?"

Monk replied in the affirmative. There he was, poor Monk, all alone on the stage, sitting on that stool like a ceramic figurine in front of all those hungry lions. They hadn't even offered him a doughnut.

Riley: "You are aware, Dr. Monk, that the administration of morphine in a patient with traumatic belly pain is contraindicated. One does not treat a symptom and **miss** the disease. One diagnoses and then intervenes. A physician doesn't offer the opiate, but not the cure, Dr. Monk. I believe Doctor Hippocrates first taught that?"

Monk explained that Pyramid, Inc. was sending him to a three-day seminar on Advanced Trauma Life Support toward the end of the month, and he would be better prepared to answer the question at that time. Rosenthal, the associate chief-of-surgery, choked on his cruller. He coughed so hard Riley almost Heimliched him.

Riley (getting hot at this point): "Dr. Rosenthal, I think we should buy Dr. Monk a handgun. A handgun, so he can plug them right there in the emergency room. I mean, there's no sense draining the blood bank, using up x-ray's film, and keeping the operating-room crew on overtime if Dr. Monk is going to kill them anyway. It just didn't make any sense. A handgun, plug them right down there in the emergency room.

Rosenthal stood up, all six-foot-three of him with his big round asymmetric face, speaking out of the right corner of his mouth.

Rosenthal: "Why not a pickup truck, Dr. Riley? Then Dr. Monk could back over them in the parking lot. That would save the expense of being seen in the emergency room in these cost conscious days. Why not send Dr. Monk out behind the paramedics? Then he could back over them at the scene and spare them the ambulance ride. Obviously, obviously, the answer is a pickup truck.

Radiologist: "We were just curious, Dr. Monk, why did you order an x-ray of the abdomen?"

Riley: "Yes, Doctor Monk, why did you order that x-ray? What were you expecting to find in the abdominal film of an unrestrained driver involved in a head-on collision, suffering left-upper-quadrant abdominal pain, and having a large black and blue mark over her left lower rib cage? What were you expecting Dr. Monk, appendicitis maybe? Gallstones? Yes, Dr. Rosenthal, for once I think we agree on something."

Poor bewildered, doughtnutless Monk sat there in a daze, clueless, his only movement being the occasional twirling of the hairs in his nose. He had been invited to Death and Doughnuts as the director of the Dupage Emergency Department, a position of respect, an honor personally bestowed upon him by Norman Lyle in Pyramid's home office, and now look at how real doctors treated him, exactly the same as before. Monk retreated to his peculiar, blank, glassy stare when befuddled. His electroencephalogram was even flatter than normal, flatter than his reduced tempo when he was diagnosing and treating emergency patients. If Rosenthal ever saw the electrocerebral silence in Monk's brain, he'd take him to surgery to donate his kidneys.

Ironically, Riley and Rosenthal had battled it out for the Chief of Surgery position for over a year in their community hospital. Neither one wanted it. They both tried to weasel out of the onerous paperwork, the administrative duties, and the complaints from nurses, other doctors, each other, aides, orderlies, janitors, cooks and God knows who else. Rosenthal won this year so Riley had to be the Chief of Surgery again.

After Death and Doughnuts, Rosenthal said to Adkins, "Who the hell would want to be the director of the emergency room anyway? And what's all this contract nonsense? I'm a surgeon, like Riley, although I do more cases than he does. We're fee for service, and would never consider working for some group a thousand miles away. I certainly wouldn't work for a group that employed over a hundred other surgeons, moving them from hospital to hospital, especially if they kept fucking up. This isn't real, is it? I certainly wouldn't give them ten to eighty per cent of my income for 'management.' I might give them five per cent if I were spared dining, never mind wining, the dopey administrator."

The mere presence of the O-J-T-er was known to exacerbate Rosenthal's hypertension.

Adkins replied, "The directorship of surgery is an unpaid position, but the groups are different. By 'managing' the emergency rooms, they receive more money than any single one of the physicians working there. That's right, and not see any patients themselves. A 'manager' of an emergency medicine group takes money out of other doctors' fees, and ends up making more money than any single physician in the group and *doesn't see any patients himself.*"

Rosenthal simply didn't believe Adkins, and as he scratched his left armpit he wanted to fire Adkins on the spot for being so misinformed, but then again, he couldn't fire Adkins since he hadn't hired him.

"Also," Adkins continued, "the group 'manages' the emergency room from a hundred or so miles away through their proxy director. Didn't Pyramid respond with the utmost of cordiality every time you disagreed with the emergency physician? When was the last time one of the orthopedists responded cordially to one of your complaints? When was the last time *you* responded cordially to someone else's complaint? And by the way, why didn't the emergency physician respond himself rather than one of the 'suits' a thousand miles away. Think about it Rosenthal. Didn't Pyramid invite you to those fancy luncheons they held? Do the neurosurgeons ever invite you to fancy lunches? To listen to your complaints? Hell's bells, no!

"If the director of the emergency room disagrees with you and you make trouble with the administrator, and the administrator complains to Pyramid, and the director says he's medically correct and won't back down, and Pyramid senses a loss of profit, what do you think will happen? The director either accepts a position at another hospital or gets fired, right? Do you think Pyramid will lose ten cents?"

"Obviously, obviously. But what about their organization, that Academy?" asked the irritated Rosenthal, his face getting more lopsided. "The American College of Surgeons virtually insists their members work independently, being personally responsibly for their own patients' care, and not giving up forty per cent of their income to some group of thugs legally protected by a corporate fiction."

Adkins said, "The American Academy of Emergency Physicians has tacitly told their members it's the groups and the contract holders or you don't work. Period. And don't make any waves."

Rosenthal was shocked, but still not fully believing this saga of pyramids of emergency medicine with the vast majority of income going to the few at the top, the few at the top who saw the least number of patients. Faced with this ethical quandary Rosenthal pulled the old surgical ploy, blaming the pathology department for everything, finally saying, "Well, look Adkins. You're the one who got Monk fired in the first place. How come you let him back?"

Adkins stared in disbelief, and was left muttering to himself, "No wonder they fired Dan Anderson."

☎

Excuse us Phoenix, but we're a bit confused. We're lay people reading this book, and you're going a bit too fast for us. Might we ask you a few questions?

Oh, yes, I'm sorry. I was concerned about my explanations on petechiae, ecchymoses, and ruptured spleens. I know I should have elaborated more.

No, no, not at all. The explanations were pretty good. It's just that, well...we're beginning to agree with Doctor Rosenthal. This story is too unbelievable. There simply can't be anything like this in American medicine, especially in something as important as emergency medicine.

Oh?

That's right, we're professionals. I'm an attorney, a graduate of Yale Law, and my husband is an accountant. We know how difficult it is to make a hundred thousand dollars a year. Surely there's no American doctor who makes a hundred thousand dollars a year for scheduling one emergency room?

You mean "managing."

Whatever! The point is, no physician takes a 20-30% cut out of the doctor's fee of the doctor who actually sees and treats my child!

Thirty per cent is low.

This doesn't exist!

That's what the "scrubs" thought.

And these "managers," the ones you call the "suits." Their main office is not really two hundred miles away. I mean the main office is not in Boston, and the "managed" emergency room somewhere outside of Buffalo?

That's a little close.

I'm warning you, Phoenix, I know lawyers. In fact, I am a lawyer. You'd better be right. If you're saying a "generic" or a Monk is seeing my child at two a.m. for the croup or, God forbid, meningitis, and thirty per cent of my physician's fee is going to a crip or a blood who is sleeping a thousand miles away, I'm going to be mighty pissed off.

You should be.

I am already undergoing a lot of intentional emotional distress because of this book.

You should be.

Wait a minute, we live in the same neighborhood as physicians.

Oh?

Yes, next door is a urologist. You mean he works for a crip or a blood?

There are no crips or bloods in urology.

All right then, on top of the hill there's an ophthalmologist. How does she make her money?

She removes cataracts.

Does she give a sizable percentage of her income to a "management" group?

There are no "management" groups in ophthalmology.

How do the orthopedists make their money?

They fix broken bones.

Which orthopedist makes the most money?

The one who repairs the most bones.

And so, the emergency physician who sees the most patients, and treats the most serious and complicated diseases makes the most money, right?

Absolutely incorrect. The one who kitchen schedules makes the most money.

I'm going to write to somebody.

There's no one to write to.

I'll write to the American Academy of Emergency Physicians.

The thumbs up their asses?

You underestimate me, Phoenix. I am the American public. I can move mountains. I will find the right people, and we will change this situation, and change it overnight. We will know right down to the penny to whom our emergency physician's fee goes, and we will cut the "suits" off at the knees. We will legislate that into every state. Are you forgetting the Emergency Medical Services System Act of 1973? It changed a lot of things overnight, didn't it, Phoenix?

Well, yes, but...

Continue on with this book. I want to see what happens to Mahoney and Steinerman, and by the way, Phoenix, you'd better be right.

I am.

CHAPTER SEVEN

CAVEAT EMPTOR

"Today's marketplace is no place to be on your own."
—*Consumer Reports, 1989*

Bing could be summed up in one phrase, he was a nice guy, a very nice guy. Bing wasn't christened "Bing," but acquired the name early in his sophomore year at the Boston Latin School when his voice changed overnight, developing a resonant, rich Bing Crosby quality.

His mannerisms also evolved—he was constantly playing Father O'Malley in *The Bells of Saint Mary's*—and it was almost uncanny to watch his choir-boy style. The nickname stuck, stuck to the point where no one in Boston actually knew Bing's real first name.

Bing had been an obstetrician-gynecologist in the Greater Boston area for seventeen years, and delivered more babies than anyone in town. He was well known to physician families, and had a long waiting list for patient acceptance. It could be said that Bing probably never sat through an entire dinner without answering a phone call.

He was a good husband and father to his three children, albeit he was guilty of the common venial sin of many physician parents, absenteeism. For many years he'd borrowed the euphemism from the pre-feminist women's movement about "quality time," which he often wondered about. One day he said to his wife aloud when the whole family was on their way to the Berkshire Mountains in their station wagon, "Has the quality time begun yet?" His children were good kids, but his son did come down with a fairly common physician's son's disease, lack of ambition.

Bing himself was growing tired, feeling modestly guilty, and looking for an honorable way out of his obstetrical and gynecologic practice. But rather than actively pursue an exit, he ended up doing what most physicians did, the exact opposite of what they really wanted, and Bing suddenly started taking welfare patients.

After reading about the lack of prenatal care in a group of lower-income women who'd recently moved into his parish, Bing horrified his office nurses by announcing that they were going to start accepting medical-assistance mothers as patients. Bing had no idea at the time he was sowing the seeds of his departure from obstetrics and gynecology.

Welfare paid the physician a flat three hundred dollars for the inclusive prenatal care and delivery of the baby, and that flat fee included monthly office visits, a sonogram, complications, delivery, and postpartum care. Bing even got one of the new, unsuspecting Catholic Filipino pediatricians to accept newborn patients for at least the first three months of life.

Pregnant welfare women were a study unto themselves, demonstrating the limitations of the maternal instinct. Bing found that two-thirds of the welfare mothers did not keep their appointments, and it bewildered Bing throughout the next few years why this was so consistent . He decided to use Thursday afternoons to schedule the appointments of the welfare mothers, and then triple booked. With only one-third of the pregnant women showing up, this scheduling arrangement worked out rather well.

What didn't work out so well was the phone. Bing's dinners were now a nightmare as he not only answered the phone, but found himself arguing with teenage girls or their mothers, often hanging up angrily, further alienating his own family. He mentioned this to some colleagues (who were not accepting welfare patients) who told Bing he didn't "train" his patients properly, and that's why they bothered him endlessly. One night a pregnant welfare patient called him from *The Sneaki Tiki* bar at 2 a.m. complaining of a headache. When Bing explained she shouldn't be drinking in the third month of pregnancy, she got rather unpleasant, threatened him with a lawsuit, and hung up.

Shortly after this event, Bing was indeed hit with a lawsuit, but it came from a different woman named Connie Thompson. Ms. Thompson had missed every prenatal appointment, except the first one, showing up in labor with contractions three minutes apart, nine centimeters dilated with a double-footling breach (feet coming out of the womb instead of the head) at the Boston Memorial Hospital, located thirty-five minutes from his office, barring traffic.

Bing left his waiting room full of patients, paying ones, and delivered a healthy baby, but the obese woman developed postpartum bleeding from a condition known as placenta accreta, a condition where the placenta, for unknown reasons, grows into the uterus, literally fingering its way deep into the uterine muscle, and the two cannot be separated after birth. There's only one alternative to maternal death in severe placenta accreta, and that is rapid hysterectomy, which is what Bing did.

Several months later, his patient, from whom he hadn't heard since, was watching the late-night movie. During the station break, an advertisement with an 800 number offered legal assistance to anyone who'd been injured by a physician, but Connie Thompson was unclear as to whether or not she'd been injured by Doctor Bing. Even though it was three a.m., actually the middle of the day for Connie, she called Bing to ask whether or not she'd been injured by him.

Bing was startled into full alertness by the third ring, since in those days all doctors owned the old AT&T phones that rang like firebells, but he was still unclear as to the nature of the call, and hung up. Connie called the 800 number which appeared for the eighth time that night on the TV screen, and the "firm" sued.

It wasn't quite the legal firm Paul Newman was up against in the movie *The Verdict*, but it was enough of a pain in the ass for the insurance company to give Connie five grand, enabling her to go on a drunken spree to Atlantic City, which all in all wasn't the best, or perhaps the worst, redistribution of monies democracy has ever seen.

Bing was furious the insurance company hadn't even contacted him, but the insurance company explained he'd signed a waiver giving the company the right to settle out of court without the physician's consent. They tried to explain to Bing this nuisance suit wasn't worth defending since Connie was simply asking for "too little," and it would cost the company twelve thousand dollars for attorney time and paper shuffling alone. It was a lose-lose situation all the way. According to the insurance company, all Bing would suffer in reality was a little smudge next to his good name, and even then, the other physicians would know the truth, and his insurance rates and insurability would not change.

Unfortunately, it did affect Bing personally, especially now that his children were getting older and less and less motivated. Because the insurance company was too lazy to defend the meritless case, the next time Bing renewed his medical license, he had to send a short "letter of explanation" to the Massachusetts Medical Society regarding his "settlement." In fact, it turned out to be a moderate-to-large sized smudge as Bing was aghast to read his name headlining the second section of the community newspaper,

ANOTHER LOCAL PHYSICIAN LOSES MALPRACTICE SUIT

"I didn't lose!" the demoralized Bing screamed on deaf ears, and the disenchanted Bing switched out of obstetrics altogether, no longer accepting public-aid patients.

Norman Lyle had long known of Bing, liked him immensely, and made Bing an offer to become a consultant in the new "quality assurance" division in Pyramid, Inc. Bing was quite grateful for the offer, and wrote a sober and moving farewell address to the *New England Journal of Medicine* explaining his "reluctant departure" from the solo, private practice of obstetrics and gynecology, which got him many spirited, sympathetic letters, and Bing never looked back.

When Lyle obtained Bing, it was an incredible coup, as Bing was so well known and liked in the Greater Boston area. Many hospital administrators personally took Bing's phone calls, and shortly after arriving at Pyramid, Inc., he called those administrators just as Lyle expected he would. But even Lyle had no idea how helpful Bing would become, how much Bing wished to become a true believer, how he would take to the constant train of euphemisms about the "mission" of Pyramid, Inc.

Bing was ferociously energetic in his job, and Lyle became suspicious he might be a second-rate spy sent in to expose Pyramid's proprietary information to Goldman. Eventually Lyle realized Bing was just tailor-made for the job, simply wanting to do the Admiral's bidding, and stay out of his own sugar frosted flakes nightmare.

Lyle saw the need for impressive physicians like Bing, and he coined a familiar term in emergency medicine: "sidekicks." "Sidekicks" were usually excellent, clinical physicians who, for whatever reasons, left their private practices, going to work for a crip or a blood, giving their organization a facade of respectability so necessary now in the competitive world of "management." Lyle was too much of a cheapskate to pay Bing a full year's salary for "quality assurance," so Bing worked in Lyle's emergency-room contract hospitals, becoming a sort of good-will ambassador. Bing also discovered how much he liked emergency medicine.

Ironically, he ended up working about the same number of hours per week as before, still getting no closer to God or family, but for unknown reasons his guilt disappeared. He enjoyed the new hospitals, the morning chats with the hospital administrators over coffee, and he enjoyed the medicine itself. He liked treating the college girls, realizing how much of emergency medicine was, in fact, primary care gynecology. He liked plastic suturing, reading cardiograms and interpreting chest x-rays. Bing's calling was to be a physician, but his true vocation was emergency medicine, a field in which he soon rose to the top, a field in the early nineteen eighties where many physicians were called, and too many were chosen.

Bing was sterling, such a natural that Lyle often used him for trouble spots. Bing would charm the patients and local physicians, buy pizza for the evening-shift nurses, and stay up and kaffeeklatsch with the overweight white women and thin Filipinos working the graveyard shifts.

Bing was sent to all new hospital contracts to give the impression he was there to stay, and that all of Pyramid's physicians were clones of the Messianic Bing, the Bing Boys. These point men that emergency medicine "management" groups initially sent to new hospital contracts were first known as "start-up" physicians, and later these true believers were called the "start-up-set-up" physicians.

Both Bing and Lyle were honest men and enjoyable guys to be around, but they formed a nefarious relationship, and together they made a treacherous pair, a two man wrecking crew, a simple bait-and-switch team that plowed many a virgin territory. It was indeed the Bings, above all the *consigliere* Bings, the well-spoken sidekicks present at all new contract negotiations, the gifted confidence men for "management," it was the Bings who became the most dangerous men in emergency medicine.

Bing was never able to work in the hospitals where he was previously on the active medical staff. He tried several times, but felt uncomfortable, deciding not to think about the many possible reasons, and choosing never to work or visit the three hospitals where he'd spent most of his adult life in his previous career (ob-gyn). Lyle once asked him about it out of curiosity, but Bing sat there, unspeaking, not knowing the reason, but unperturbed by the question. He simply said, "You don't put new wine into old wineskins." Bing said it because he couldn't articulate the real reason, but Lyle found the quote brilliantly appropriate, never asking again. Lyle and Bing left the office early that night for they needed a good night's rest. Tomorrow was a big day for them at Braintree Children's Hospital.

Steinerman also had one of those feeling, and was also not able to articulate it—but something wasn't quite right. It was a sense of not belonging, and the next morning, Steinerman complained about it to Mahoney. It was early, and Mahoney was only half-listening while Steinerman mulled over this vague notion as they drove.

Lyle had invited both Mahoney and Steinerman to the contract negotiation session with the administrator of the Braintree Children's Hospital. The hospital administrator had taken Lyle's bait, responding to the promises in the fancy glossies mailed from Pyramid, Inc. What Steinerman and Mahoney didn't know, was Lyle had told the administrator he was bringing along two prototypical physicians who worked for Pyramid, Inc., who were also considering working at Braintree. Lyle had simply told Steinerman and Mahoney to wear suits for the luncheon because the restaurant they were going to required jackets.

Meanwhile, Lyle was up bright and early, beginning the important day at the Hancock Building, preparing for the frontal assault on the hospital administrator of Braintree Children's Hospital.

His delta force included two of his best looking marketers with charts and graphs, Bing, and Valerie Longo. Lyle checked his well-scripted men and women himself, like a five star general with all the heavy responsibilities. Not only must everyone's apparel match, but the group must not clash with each other in any other way, and particularly their colognes and perfumes. He went through the spiel of Operation Braintree like a true craftsman, making sure the "sidekick" Bing knew by heart the position the marketers had designed, and how the reality of this emergency medicine "management" group and their motives had to be precisely and perfectly blurred as they prepared using a host of old Hollywood techniques.

There was only one gold medal in emergency medicine "management," no silver, no bronze. Lyle knew the gold would be won by a desperately thin margin, and he had to instill a win-at-all-costs attitude. Their main message was pure theater distilled in the glitz of charts and graphs presented by good looking, well-tailored young men and women who were themselves tailoring the message to the unwitting O-J-T-er. "The medium is the message," and it was to be delivered by the masters of manipulation, à la emergency medicine. Lyle went over the strategic analysis again and again with his co- expeditionists to make sure his presentation was better than any of the other six piranha vying for this jackpot. He knew the presentations to most of the O-J-T-ers amounted to little more than a crapshoot, and if he hit one wrong button, the crips would get the lucrative quarry of the kitchen scheduling contract.

The assassination squad arrived at exactly thirteen hundred hours. The poor O-J-T-er was simply outclassed by the lighthearted Bing, the warmhearted Valerie Longo paying lip service to patient advocacy, the chartsy-graphsy couple, and the authoritarian Lyle. After the well-choreographed presentation at the hospital, the Pyramid legation took the mudhead O-J-T-er out to lunch at the finest restaurant in Needham, where they ordered Maine lobster accompanied by a Robert Mondavi Chardonnay. Smooth as silk Bing took the liberty of ordering the wine, as every successful emergency medicine "management" group had their own sommelier whose job was to suggest a wine before the O-J-T-er ordered something unpotable. No one wanted the hospital administrator nervous at any point, especially fumbling with a wine list, unable to pronounce the various varietals in front of him.

From their ringside seats, Mahoney and Steinerman, as usual, watched in awe, knowing they had so much proprietary information to learn. In fact, at this age, it might be hopeless since the bottomless pit of proprietary information was something one had to learn at an early age, like gymnastics or languages. If only they hadn't wasted so much time completing their residencies.

The fare arrived. Steinerman was impressed when the silver dome of his plate was removed revealing a very substantial crustacean; Valerie had made excellent arrangements. But he gasped when the white-gloved, tuxedoed waiter removed the silver dome from the O- J-T-er's plate. Even Lyle was taken aback as the hospital administrator stared at the Loch Ness Monster in front of him. It was so big they all hoped Pyramid hadn't done anything illegal.

They ate and drank and roared with laughter while the O-J-T-er almost ruined dinner with his chuckleheaded humor. After the squad had created the necessary fireside warmth, Lyle began his benediction. His baritone voice was lowered an octave as he spoke of the seriousness of their mission, "to put together the finest emergency-medical-care team. Together we'll do it, and as a team, we can make this hospital's emergency department a flagship...," pausing as he looked straight at the O-J-T-er through his blue-tinted Baush and Lomb contact lenses, powerphrasing him with, "...possibly the finest emergency room on the east coast."

The assassination squad nodded their heads solemnly, and even the O-J-T-er consensually nodded with reverence as the word "team" kept perseverating through his mind. Lyle had such a fine way to fine tune the communication to capture the essence of what the administrator needed to hear, and the O-J-T-er had heard "team" in his night-school course in administration, and he liked it.

"Team, team," he kept repeating to himself like a mantra, "as a team..."

With the prowess of Olivier, Lyle lowered his voice yet another octave as the Iago of emergency medicine ended the soliloquy with the magic words as only the gospel-inflected Norman Lyle could recite them; *Yes, Mr. Hospital Administrator, the bottom line of our group is quality.*

There was a heavy silence in the room, even at nearby tables. The O-J-T-er sensed his big break in life—to become associated with this well-dressed group of charming magicians—and he wanted to make his emergency-medical-care team a well "managed" group, the finest snake oil on the east coast. With no sign of a painful struggle, he Dan Andersoned himself and his hospital onto the dotted line. He would get Bing to staff his emergency room for the first six probationary weeks, and then Lyle would kick the poor bastard in the balls with Monk and Walsh.

Although Valerie had worn extra tampons, her vaginal vault was so full it began to smell up the whole restaurant. Mahoney had a sense of puzzlement on his face while that vaguely familiar acrid smell permeated the air. Steinerman recognized the quizzical look on his friend's face, and handed him a folded note under the table. Mahoney unfolded it, and looking at the word, now recognized the smell, t-r-i-c-h-o-m-o-n-a-s.

After the homicide, Bing had to go home to take a nap since he was working the night shift, and Valerie had to work in the ICU at Boston Children's. It was still early in the day, so Lyle asked Mahoney and Steinerman to accompany him to the Hancock building. They agreed, and for sport, Lyle took the bedazzled physicians for a privileged look into the inner sanctum, the fifth floor "war room." Entering the two story room, Mahoney and Steinerman stared at the incredible electronic map occupying the facing wall, a huge map of the entire northeast corridor with different colored small lights on it referred to as "pins." Each pin represented a hospital with an active emergency room.

Steinerman and Mahoney stood frozen, thinking they'd just entered NORAD. They thought they were in the middle of a Colorado mountain or were cast as extras in the movie *War Games.* They saw a dozen people in front of computer terminals, like NASA before a launch. The mind-boggled Steinerman started to speak slowly like he was scared (Mahoney couldn't speak at all), and finally stuttered, "Norman, what do the different colored lights on this map signify?"

One of the techs at the computer started explaining, "The green lights represent hospitals where we already have the contracts so we don't call their administrators. In fact, we're not allowed to talk to them at all. The yellow pins represent established contracts of other groups, especially five-to-fifteen member, board-accredited physician groups, usually stable, and we don't waste an excessive amount of time on them. However, we do know the expiration date of every emergency room contract in their 'region,' and when the renewal times of their contracts come up, we change the yellow pins to red pins."

Surprisingly, Lyle let the tech go on airing proprietary information. "Red pins also signify emergency medicine contracts having 'windows of vulnerability,' maybe a disgruntled administrator or an antagonistic staff physician wanting to change the 'management' group. This is one of the 'services' we provide, and we call the hospitals represented by the red pins on a regular and frequent basis," the tech said to the two catatonic figures in front of him.

Apparently, Pyramid, Inc. had sources everywhere, "windows" representing crucial information. There were a lot of barracudas in the emergency medicine contract "management" tank so the crips had to get there before the bloods scooped the brass ring. The techs spent their entire working day calling the O-J-T-ers of the "red pin" hospitals.

Lyle had gone to the men's room, and now rejoined Steinerman and Mahoney. He looked at the school children completely awed by this massive enterprise, in a state of stupefaction, and suddenly felt that recurrent contempt in the pit of his gut. The "scrubs" learned cardiograms and trauma, toxicology and plastic suturing, meningitis and antibiotics, but they didn't know a damn thing about "management." These tinhorns didn't even have their own corporations, they weren't presidents of anything, and Lyle had to all but contain his urge to send these two pitiable clinicians out to the luncheonette to fetch him some coffee. The kitchen schedulers had come a long way, and emergency medicine "management" had become a very lucrative bitch in this high-tech era.

As Lyle looked upward, he suddenly saw through the techs on the sixth floor, pledge drivers on high, the red and yellow pin departments in the middle, crips and bloods, sidekicks everywhere. It was an incredible vision as all of a sudden Lyle saw the roof of the Hancock building open, open into Michelangelo's heaven, and Lyle for a brief moment saw God, and realized God was no Mahoney or Steinerman. God didn't read cardiograms or treat croup or differentiate diaper rashes, God was an entrepreneur who held many contracts, a CEO, a "suit," a man with a degree but few clinical skills, a man with trillions of hours of "management" services, and while Lyle was having a vision more significant than Lourdes, his trance was abruptly broken by the sight of those two utility infielders, Mahoney and Steinerman. For the first time in his life, Lyle felt like he might fit somewhere, somewhere but not of this world, and Norman Lyle was thankful to God above he was not a Catholic or a Jew, but an ill-fitting transcendentalist who had built this majestic cathedral in honor of the God of the emergency medicine marketplace, the one true God.

After the cook's tour, Lyle guided the dazed Mahoney and Steinerman out of the Hancock Building, feeling like a seeing-eye dog helping the two of them across the street. Full of mirth, he took them to the local watering hole for a few beers, mainly to gloat a little longer in such distinguished company.

Unfortunately, Jonathan Stullman was there. Everyone in Boston hated the Stullmans, a dynasty of three generations of gonzo orthopedic surgeons from Beacon Hill who had close to a one-hundred-year educational history at the Johns Hopkins University, and no one ever knew why the Doctor Great Great Grandfather Stullman had left Baltimore, inflicting his lineage on Boston. Steinerman remembered when his grandfather died, Stullman's father came to pay his respects, and on his way out, Doctor Stullman left a stack of his business cards next to the registration book.

Jonathan Stullman was a pure and proud Stullman, a sociopath who'd found his niche in life in the field of kitchen scheduling. Stullman wanted to stay an up and coming con man, but his father wouldn't hear of it, and after much family wrangling, Stullman announced he was going to begin his orthopedic residency training at the Hopkins. Stullman was on his way out, but joined them for a beer, although all three of them would have gladly disinvited him. But old Stullman had some pretty big news of his own. His eight hospital "management" contracts, all golden gooses which were putting seventy-five grand apiece clear profit into his back pocket annually, were astonishingly enough, up for sale. Even Lyle gasped.

"Up for sale?" replied the shocked Lyle. Who ever heard of a kitchen scheduler's contract up for sale he wondered? Lyle joked, "Well, I'll give you a hundred bucks for each one. Eight hundred bucks for the bunch, take it or leave it."

Stullman chuckled, "Try fifty thousand each, maybe for you Norman, three hundred and fifty thou for the whole bunch."

Lyle, Mahoney, and Steinerman didn't know how to react, whether to laugh or gasp.

"That's right, fifty thousand smackers each, that's what Goldman is willing to pay."

They all just stared.

"Well, think about it Norman. My taxi meter never stops, I'm making twenty dollars an hour at each hospital, all clear profit, twenty-four hours a day, seven days a week, fifty-two fat weeks a year. I actually make more money when I'm sleeping, and that all adds up to a pretty nice chunk of change for a good old country boy like me (the family had a vacation home in the Berkshires). I think those contracts are a steal at fifty."

Lyle got uncomfortable with Stullman's fanfare because he didn't like the "scrubs" knowing how much he was skimming off the top for "managing," especially the amount he made when he was sleeping.

Stullman got up to leave, parting with, "Think about it Norman. I'd rather sell 'em to you than that jerkoff Goldman."

Stullman walked out, and the three sat there staring at one another until Mahoney said, "That can't be, can it?"

Lyle quickly stuttered, "Oh no. No. He's well, Stullman's just a blow hard. There's no way he could be selling emergency medicine contracts. I mean, they don't have any value. The hospital wouldn't allow such a thing. He's lying. Besides, Goldman's no fool. He wouldn't buy an abstraction. Administrating an emergency room 'management' contract is hard work. What does Stullman think, I'm Tom Sawyer?"

They continued to drink, made a few strained jokes, and Lyle abruptly excused himself. He was pondering, needing to take a long drive, a long think drive. "Could this be true?"

But then it started to make more and more sense to him. At twenty dollars an hour for scheduling, he saw that in just one year he could make close to double his money back. In two years, he would have an extremely handsome return on his investment. By the time he'd driven to Gloucester, he'd realized Stullman was offering a damn good deal.

Stullman would have to sell the physician noncompete clauses with the "management" contracts, and not tell the hospitals the parent company would be Pyramid, Inc. "managing" them. One of the hospitals was St. Ann's, Lyle's Kittyhawk, and another was St. Joseph's, Dan Anderson's old hospital, and neither one would let Pyramid, Inc. back on a bet.

Lyle could form a dummy corporation with Stullman swearing secrecy about the aliases. Stullman could even sell him all his company stock in the same "management" group's name so the hospitals wouldn't even have to know the corporate shells had changed hands. He could then hire Stullman back as a consultant, making Stullman sign a legally-binding letter of secrecy.

Lyle, the CEO, was getting rather excited, seeing how Pyramid, Inc. could expand by block-buying the "management" contracts of other kitchen schedulers.

The "managed" emergency rooms could then be directed from the war room, and different colored pins could describe possible takeovers. Lyle, the staunch champion of central planning, envisioned the next Great Leap Forward for Pyramid, Inc. He could seize the wealth by sniffing around, looking for brewing takeovers along with his one-by-one acquisitions.

Another market was suddenly born as Lyle thought, "Commodities. Yes. Like coffee, corn, or soybeans, emergency-room 'management' contracts can be bought and sold on the open market. I've got to call Stullman as soon as I get home. Stupid Stullman, he's undervalued his commodities. The free market system," the jubilant Lyle thought. "My God," yelping aloud like a puppy dog, "the free market system!"

The energetic Lyle was full of stamina and purpose, on the phone as soon as he got home, but his heart sank when Stullman told him he'd already completed the deal with Goldman, the usually impervious Lyle gasping again.

Lyle hung up thinking, "Maybe Goldman has some cash flow problems. After all, he's just taken on a pretty hefty debt."

Norman had to slow down. He didn't want to waste time, but he also didn't want to give Goldman the impression he was panic buying. He knew Stullman had demanded cash. Goldman's treasury might be depleted by a four-hundred-thousand-dollar outlay, and this could be an opportune time to make an offer. Maybe the swashbuckling Goldman had over-extended, suffocating under a mountain of acquisition-related debt, needing to sell one or two contracts at a small loss? Lyle dialed slowly, then asked Goldman if he might want to sell a contract or two of Stullman's.

Goldman said "Sure," but there was only one catch—the wily Goldman was far from liquidation. Goldman realized, as well, that Stullman had sold at bargain-basement prices, and he offered Lyle two of the kitchen scheduling contracts—each one for the asking price of one-hundred-and-twenty-five thousand dollars.

The crestfallen Lyle gasped again, but this time he'd done the arithmetic. He knew he couldn't leave the offer on the table, and choked while he said, "Fine, I'll cut the check and meet with you tomorrow."

CHAPTER EIGHT

CRO-MAGNON

"Surgery does the ideal thing,
it separates the patient from the disease."
—*Clendening*

Steinerman's father was a rheumatologist from the south end of Boston, and his partner was Neil Sugarman, a gastroenterologist. They shared an office with all of its encumbrances, the x-ray machine, a centrifuge for separating blood elements, salaries of the help, rent, the phone, etc. They split their earnings at the end of the year, and never nickeled or dimed each other about who actually grossed what, their partnership continuing for twelve years. Both of them saw many "general practice" type patients, but Doctor Steinerman received more referrals than Sugarman.

Sugarman was a so-so gastroenterologist, but most physicians didn't refer their ulcers, gallstones, or colon bleeds in the nineteen fifties and sixties to a gastroenterologist. There were a limited number of treatment options available back then, and when things didn't work, the internists simply sent their patients to a surgeon who would deal with the dilemma definitively, following the guidelines of the surgical dictum, "When in doubt, cut it out."

Physicians did, however, refer to Doctor Steinerman. They

referred their rheumatoid arthritis, lupus, intractable gout, and if they could, the nebulous chronic joint pains, neck aches, and lower back problems the orthopedists refused to see. Steinerman's dad was a bit of a softie, his secretaries never asking about insurance policies or previous referrals.

But a rheumatologist cannot part the patients from their diseases. Rheumatology is a demanding profession requiring an extra allotment of time for the support of both patient and family. Many forms of arthritis are relentlessly progressive and debilitating diseases, and drug therapy has to be individualized, tailor made after a frustrating period of trial and error using drug combinations of varying dosages. In the nineteen seventies an explosion of anti-inflammatory medications appeared, and along with them a laundry list of side effects, side effects which many rheumatologists and their patients learned the hard way, the Doctor Westerly way. Both Doctors Steinerman and Sugarman worked long hours in an unenviable lifestyle for their hundred grand a year.

Doctors Steinerman and Sugarman taught medical students at two University medical schools, and many of their former students referred cases to them, mostly to Doctor Steinerman and occasionally to Sugarman. Neil Sugarman wasn't the brightest doctor alive, and physically had a minor defect—a small forehead. It wasn't just a small one, but a very small forehead, one that a phrenologist might take notes on. Actually his forehead was so small, the medical students, interns, and residents referred to Doctor Sugarman as Cro-Magnon, and for short, everyone called him Cro, although never to his face. Cro also had large white teeth, and when he smiled broadly, many people found themselves thinking of Cheetah. It was considered a fortunate thing that Richard Leaky never saw Cro walking down the street because Leakey would have commandeered that cranium to the anthropology department for study. Cro soldiered on though, and saw patients with the full gamut of stomach and bowel diseases. He dressed well, spoke all right, and was a reasonable, if somewhat dull-witted, fellow. Being associated with Doctor Steinerman was the tide Cro needed to raise his boat.

However, in the mid-sixties, an incredible event occurred. A funny flashlight was developed, covered by a flexible rubber tube, a light that could bend around corners, a light that could slip down an esophagus, sliding into the stomach, allowing the viewer to see with his or her naked eye the stomach and the duodenum, a light that could slip up the anus, through the sigmoid, up the descending colon, around the flexure of the spleen, looping by the liver impression as the light peered into one's innards.

This flashlight replaced many of the limitations of clinical evaluation and x-ray contrast studies because non-surgical physicians could actually see ulcers for the first time, along with polyps, cancers, pus, and bleeding sites.

A new star was born in medicine, and it was made to shine as one of the most interesting and easiest high-tech medical procedures also became one of the most expensive in all of internal medicine. All physicians were informed of this by *the fat man* in *The House of God* who said, "There's a fortuna in shit."

When the flashlight initially came out, Cro-Magnon went to an introductory seminar, and was one of the first physicians in Boston to actually purchase fiber optics. He suddenly became the physician most in demand in the Boston medical community, with hospitals calling him around the clock to slide his flashlight up or down a body hollow.

The beleaguered Cro was given emergency one-day privileges in many hospitals just to bring his flashlight in to look into the gullets and colons of his many referrals who were literally lined up in front of the emergency room, where he performed his procedures in those days.

Month after month his gastroenterology payments dwarfed Doctor Steinerman's rheumatology checks. In the first year of the new light, without any misuse, Cro-Magnon grossed four hundred and seven thousand dollars, and so he did what he had to do. He went to Doctor Steinerman and told him, after twelve years, they were no longer partners. He was moving out of the office, and move he did.

Cro not only moved out of the office, but moved out of Boston altogether to North Adams where he became the chairman of the newly-created department of Gastroenterology, a medical specialty hardly existing less than a year before, chief at the Berkshire Community Hospital, the department having only one member, Cro-Magnon.

Truth be known, no one really missed Cro, although Doctor Steinerman felt bad at first since they were partners for so long, and it was just the money unilaterally splitting them up. Long after, he felt Cro should have just approached him with a new arrangement, but didn't know at the time Cro was afraid Doctor Steinerman would be angry. In fact, Cro had preemptively moved to North Adams because somewhere in his paranoid brainstem he thought Doctor Steinerman was already bad mouthing him in the old neighborhood.

During their twelve years together, Doctor Steinerman and Cro-Magnon always enjoyed a very satisfactory set of relationships with other physicians, especially the surgeons, ophthalmologists, and cardiologists—in fact, all the medical and surgical subspecialists. Orthopedic surgeons now were perfecting total-joint replacements for patients with rheumatoid arthritis, actually beginning to separate the patient from his or her disease. Doctor Steinerman referred his patients to them regularly.

Cro also referred to the general surgeons when he obtained positive cytologies for stomach or colon cancers, and in the early days, he referred a great number of patients with bleeding ulcers, and those with intractable pain from their peptic ulcer disease.

Cro received many cases of French and California wines and bottles of his favorite, unblended scotch whiskeys over the holiday periods from the grateful surgeons to whom he referred patients. The wines decreased in number and quality after the development of a drug called cimetidine better known by its trade name, Tagamet.

Tagamet blocked the production of stomach acid, thereby reducing the pain from peptic ulcers, the bleeding, and the number of referrals to the general surgeons, reducing their income by an estimated one-fifth.

Cro-Magnon's magnums and his cases of holiday scotch dropped even further when another new tool was developed for the cave man, a pair of forceps that fit into his flashlight, enabling him to remove polyps from the colon through the flashlight. Again, the general surgeon saw income from another cause of major abdominal operations evaporate.

But since the patients were living longer, they created a larger revenue base for other specialists. Indeed, the old folks in Massachusetts couldn't see or pee as well as they used to, their bones were more brittle, snapping more frequently, and some of the old gals even wanted to know the "best plastic surgeon in town."

So the internists and general practitioners remained popular with many subspecialists within the medical community, forming the heart and soul of a symbiotic set of universal relationships existing in the private practice of medicine—except for one specialty, emergency medicine.

There was never a good reason for most physicians to hear from the emergency doctor. It almost never represented the kind of referral the staff physician wanted to get, and it was the simple nature of the crime, emergency physicians ground the gears of the referral system

Possibly an emergency patient had an allergic reaction to a recently-prescribed medication. Perhaps it was a blatant treatment failure, or maybe the patient ruptured an aortic aneurysm at two p.m. on Sunday afternoon, just prior to the kickoff of Super Bowl Sunday. Maybe the patient was in shock due to bleeding from the arthritis medicines, with a hovering family at the bedside screaming for "their doctor."

Usually the calls from the emergency room arrived after

hours or on weekends, many times regarding uninsured patients, or non-paying trauma victims who had a fearsome record of suing. Possibly the call involved a very sick patient who wanted to switch doctors, switch to the doctor on call that Saturday or Sunday making him or her a captive of the manipulative patient. The most common reason the emergency physician was calling another physician was because his or her name was on a mandatory, backup call list publicly posted in the emergency department.

The role of the emergency physician was in sharp contrast to the other staff physicians, an adversarial role, their calls to be avoided rather than embraced. Several normally-responsible doctors in every hospital regularly played hide-and-seek with their answering services when they sensed the incoming phone call was from the emergency department. Even Doctor Steinerman was caught one day low-crawling by the emergency room while entering the hospital. One night when Mahoney called the internist on the mandatory call list, the internist's five year old son yelled to his father, "Daddy, it's the goddamn E.R. doc."

Doctor Steinerman was also not pleased with Philip Mahoney or Abraham for choosing to practice emergency medicine. When Mahoney finished the residency program in emergency medicine, Doctor Steinerman was still furious with him for doing it. After medical school he had brought Mahoney into his office, and for over an hour spoke like a Dutch Uncle, telling him, "You don't go to a three year training program just to become a moonlighter, Philip! I don't understand why you are setting your sights so low?" However, the stubborn Mahoney persisted, and now Abraham, much to Doctor Steinerman's chagrin, was also doing emergency medicine full-time.

Doctor Steinerman never did hear directly from Cro, but heard at the medical-society meetings that Cro had dialed into the saturated fat crowd in North Adams and was quite prosperous with his new light.

Shortly after he moved, Cro noted something new in his own

personality as for the first time in his life he'd become somewhat abusive to other physicians, sensing they had a certain envy of his flashlighting money, which they did.

Cro learned, however, the boundaries of his referral base as he became a physician who was referred to rather than a physician who referred, and every holiday he bought the liquor rather than received it. He soon learned most family practitioners and general internists would rather their patients succumb than send them to an arrogant asshole consultant, and, in fact, many were buying shorter versions of the new flashlights themselves. Cro soon realized, like all private-practice physicians who receive referrals, that a different set of table manners was to be accorded, and so gentlemanly Cro was to the primary-care doctors. Cro's physician abusiveness then found a focus in the emergency department where he became a royal pain in the ass to many of the transient physicians who worked there.

Cro also developed an obsession, a fondness for the under-secretary to the secretary of the medical staff, the incomparably beautiful Emily Spurlock, a twenty-one year old piece of pure pulchritude dazzling anyone who saw her. Cro was fifty-seven now, and had never thought nor cared about that so called "torch" that had to be "passed to a new generation of Americans." He thought his money and position within the microcosm were powerful aphrodisiacs, like his RX-7. He assumed Emily and her rather good looking friends actually talked about and desired him, and he viewed their respectful "Good morning, Doctor" as a burning within them, a burning like the one he had for Emily, an obsessive burning as he visited Emily every day for over an hour in her office staring at her blue-green eyes. Emily occasionally complained to the medical staff secretary she couldn't get her work done, but the med-staff secretary reassured Emily, suggesting she simply chat with Cro even as his visits grew longer and longer. Emily didn't dislike Cro, just found him boring.

The hospital administration certainly didn't want Cro offended because Cro did his flashlighting in the hospital rather than the recently erected ambulatory care center the other physicians built, but wouldn't let Cro invest in because they feared the height of his forehead, many of the doctors wondering if Cro were entirely human. The hospital lost a great deal of revenue when the Surgi-Center opened because many procedures formerly done in the hospital were now done in the outpatient center. The bean-counting CPAs recognized on the hospital's monthly balance sheet that Cro-Magnon utilized the procedure room of the hospital more than anyone else, and the poorly-paid Emily Spurlock, not getting all her work done every day, was a small price to pay for it.

Although he was basically an idiot, Cro served his hospital on the emergency medicine committee, keeping a hand in who was hired to staff the emergency room. He'd met with Goldman, Lyle, and the various bunko men in Boston. Cro liked their pandering, especially enjoying the Beluga and Dom Perignon dinners, feeling a certain sense of entitlement to it.

At one contract negotiating session, Goldman tried to explain the nuances of the EMS (emergency medical services) law to Cro, but Cro blankly stared asking, "What's emergency medicine got to do with multiple sclerosis?"

Lyle and Goldman stared for a minute before minimizing Cro's vast, black hole of information, confusing EMS with MS. Both quickly sized up Cro, kid gloving him on any hard facts, but not knowing just how far down the evolutionary tree they had to go with this simian for "effective communication." Lyle and Goldman desperately wanted to be the plantation owners of the Berkshire Community Hospital emergency medicine "management" contract, but they had to depend on the administrator and this peculiar missing link who'd for some unknown reason interjected himself into the negotiations.

Surprisingly enough, and for no apparent reason, Lyle won out. Cro superciliously explained his incoherent reasoning to Goldman, who listened attentively with concealed disappointment, but taking notes knowing that Lyle would fuck up the "management" contract within a year or two. Lyle, of course, sent Bing, and had another ace up his sleeve because Philip Mahoney was looking for a job. Since Lyle had recently become the biggest mogul of emergency medicine job opportunities in Massachusetts, Mahoney was forced to work for Lyle. Things were certainly looking quite rosy for the ever-expanding base of Pyramid, Inc. in North Adams.

Cro-Magnon dozed off softly that night, realizing he'd made a Solomonic decision in securing the best "management" group to staff the Berkshire Community Hospital, never realizing the direct connection of flexible fiber optics to money and power.

As he dozed more deeply, he dreamt of those fluorescent blue-green eyes, and the young, firmly-breasted body of a woman who was almost certainly dreaming of him as well.

CHAPTER NINE

THE QUIET ROOM

"The hand is second only to the eye."
—*Aristotle*

Within six hours of arriving at the Berkshire Community Hospital in North Adams, Philip Mahoney had Emily Spurlock in the "quiet room."

The quiet room in most hospitals is sequestered out of view of the emergency room, a small, nicely-appointed area where families are taken to be told bad news. Of all hospital areas, the quiet room is the most exciting and dangerous to fornicate in since the wooden doors are large, churchlike, and don't have any locks. Emily was unusually loud when she came, and the security guard was unclear on what to do. Before the day was out, the news had been secretly leaked to Cro six independent times, including once on his new fax machine, hospital gossip traveling slightly faster than the speed of light.

Cro, whose obsession classified him as a kind of Emily "stalker," had a somewhat predictable reaction when he found out about Philip Mahoney's interlude. It was no longer business as usual with Norman Lyle and Pyramid, Inc. as Cro turned tense and red, and although no one knew the medical term for it, his entire deconditioned body actually swelled, almost physically exploding like a noodle bomb. He stormed down to the emergency room to confront the degenerate Mahoney, but Mahoney's shift had ended, and Walsh was there pinch hitting for the overstretched Bing. Cro was livid, and had his ears been younger and better he would have heard Emily since Mahoney had her again in the quiet room after Walsh relieved him. Cro might have gone over to the quiet room to hear a little "bad news," *the horror* hitting yet again in the newest medical specialty.

Lyle was amused by Mahoney but knew he had to get him out of North Adams. The sexual affairs of emergency physicians were one of the biggest "management" problems of contract groups, many times requiring the crips and bloods to board midnight airplane flights without a fourteen-day advance notice, traveling thousands of miles to sooth ruffled feathers, all paid for of course by monies taken out of the fees of the physicians actually seeing and treating the patients in the emergency rooms of the nation.

Lyle spoke directly to Cro, expressing his, "shock at such appalling, and to say the least, unprofessional behavior." Lyle said, "very stern, in-house disciplinary action will be taken," assuring Cro he was capable of meting out some pretty harsh measures.

"After this, Doctor Mahoney is going to have trouble finding work anywhere. We're going to play this one right by the book," Lyle somberly concluded with the enraged Cro.

Lyle had to quickly slam his office door shut when his new secretary Rene burst out laughing. When he hung up, he told Rene to call Bekins Van Lines to move Mahoney's belongings again.

"But Doctor Lyle, we just moved Doctor Mahoney's belongings last week," Rene giggled, but amusement was in short supply lately at Pyramid, Inc.

"Rene, please just do it."

"Yes Doctor Lyle."

Again, the Bekins money would come out of the fees of the physicians seeing and treating patients in the emergency rooms.

Lyle wondered what to do for he knew Mahoney was quick tempered, but he had to get Mahoney out of North Adams. He couldn't risk a direct confrontation, because Mahoney might then go to work for Goldman, and Lyle knew if he pissed Mahoney off, Steinerman would tell him to go fly a kite as well. Steinerman's father would also bad-mouth him in Beacon Hill, where Lyle and the former Carolyn Skanks had just bought and moved into Doctor Francis Peabody's old house.

It would be ideal for Lyle to move Mahoney to his contract hospital at Holyoke Methodist, but that was so close that Cro would find out about it. Then again, Monk had been at Holyoke for the past three months, and Lyle knew Pyramid, Inc. would be getting a call from the Holyoke O-J-T-er soon. He could practice a little prophylactic medicine by getting Monk out of there before they threw him out by simply switching Mahoney for Monk. No, he thought, Holyoke is way too close to North Adams, and Mahoney would keep fucking Emily, especially if he knew it annoyed Cro. Maybe he could temporarily move Mahoney to Cape Cod Community Hospital where one of his marketers had just busted a Goldman contract for summertime emergency-room coverage. Lyle needed some new start-up-set-up physicians, especially since the Bing Boys were completely booked. Lyle slumped there realizing yet again he was worth every penny of his income because emergency medicine "management" was such a fucking complicated bitch. Lyle suddenly remembered something.

"Rene."

"Yes, Doctor Lyle."

"Rene, call Doctor Mahoney and tell him we need to have a photo taken of him by the South Street Photographers. Make sure you tell him it's at our expense, and let him know he'll get copies. I'll explain it all to him later." Lyle couldn't talk to anyone at the moment, least of all Mahoney.

"Yes, Doctor Lyle."

Emily Spurlock had been married at sixteen, usual for a rural woman, especially the type from which men simply couldn't avert their eyes. She married a dull-witted but good-looking farmer, actually more of a farmhand on his father's orchard. Her "child" husband, like his "child" dad, was a wife-beater. Since neither one knew any other way to live, it was acceptable to the beautiful, although slightly chubby Emily, acceptable until she was browsing through the library shelves one day, because her husband stopped giving her the money to buy Harlequin romance novels, another action in his systematic attempts to make their days as lifeless and joyless as possible. Scanning through the shelves, she searched for the biggest novel she could find in case her husband forbade her to go back to the library, and at the suggestion of the fiftyish woman librarian, Emily checked out *Anna Karenina.*

She read for two straight days, virtually neglecting the constant demands of her husband, and she suffered a few ecchymotic blemishes for it, but when she finished, she knew Tolstoy was a great writer, knew he was a great writer because Emily wasn't quite putting two and two together. She also snuck out to see the movie, *Anna Karenina* when it played at Smith College. She next took out *War and Peace*, but the book seemed endless, and by the time she'd finished she was exhausted, had another purple blotch inflicted on her left cheek, and felt like she'd fought the damn Franco-Prussian war. She was halfway through *Resurrection* when she realized that she was "Anna." *Anna Karenina* was the biography of Emily Spurlock, only written by Uncle Leo over a hundred years ago, and she was living in rural North Adams, another name for pre-revolutionary Russia. She saw herself like Anna, laying down on the railroad tracks in front of the oncoming train at the end of her thirties to finally achieve the only possible relief from the oppression, the boredom of a narrow-minded, stupid and everpresent, suffocating husband, and what Flannery O'Conner called the "barbarousness of mediocrity."

After she interpreted Tolstoy correctly, she returned the unfinished *Resurrection* to the library, left her dolt of a hubby, fled might be a better term, evading his posse long enough to file the necessary papers.

Miraculously, she had remained childless up to this point, a fortuitous coming together of the stars and Catholic rhythms, and she was a tall, beautiful, good-natured young woman with striking iridescent, blue-green eyes and long, silky, brown hair. She was noninfectious and dependent-free—full of cognitive skills to boot—ready to wine, dine, rock and roll, and run off to Cape Cod with Philip Mahoney.

As a general rule, male physicians undermarry, but Emily turned out to be a real sleeper, and had no trouble getting Mahoney to put the ring on her finger. Philip couldn't take his eyes off of Emily, her blue-green, turquoise eyes keeping him almost hypnotized. Her chestnut-brown hair was now waist length and the divorce diet gave her a slender, tanned body that was so sexually responsive she came within seconds of his touch. The color of those eyes he'd seen only once before in nature, they were the color of Emerald Bay on the western shore of Lake Tahoe, a color only present about an hour after sunrise when the water was so clear one could see the bottom thirty feet below the surface. Only that water and Emily Spurlock's eyes were that blue-green sort of off-turquoise color not found anywhere else within the prism of the visible light spectrum. Mahoney nicknamed her "Tahoe" and from then on, everyone referred to Emily Spurlock as "Tahoe."

They rented a saltbox on the sand dunes and quite literally lived happily ever after, although somewhat bombastically so. When they drank, the two of them were a most amusing couple to be around, especially when their arguments escalated to Virginia Woolf intensity, punctuated with belly laughter and repartee too funny to ignore. It was an unforgettable summer for the both of them with Tom-Boy Tahoe releasing twenty-four years of pent up wildness and repressed energy.

Philip also spent time reading and writing on some unfinished toxicology papers from his days at the Hershey Medical Center, and Emily got a part-time position as a lab assistant drawing bloods.

A good audience makes a successful raconteur, and Tahoe couldn't get enough of the daily stories of the busy emergency room from Philip, stories of the patients and the mischief they got themselves into during their vacations.

Mahoney got a keen sense of the importance of an emergency room like Cape Cod Community during the summertime, when the population swelled from 165,000 to 600,000, a place where most everybody was on vacation, and away from their family physicians and referral networks. Since the local physicians were reluctant to establish short-term doctor-patient relationships in malpractice-ridden Massachusetts, where could the summer visitors turn if they found themselves in a pickle?

Obviously, obviously.

Indeed, the emergency physician represented the tip of the spear of the health care system, seeing an unscheduled, unrestricted patient population from pediatrics to geriatrics, wounded in either mind or body, an incredible lifeboat available twenty-four hours a day with (hopefully) unvarying quality. The emergency physician also tripwired the response of the patients' diseases to the subspecialists, for example, an ophthalmologist for an open eye injury or a neurosurgeon for a blood clot oppressing the brain. The patients who came to the emergency room were generally at the most vulnerable moments in their lives, *in extremis,* with simply too much to consider, some peeking for the first time into the valley of the shadow of death. These patients, now referred to as the "consumers of the health care dollar," also had to see a strange doctor, exacerbating the credibility gap.

As the roll of the memory-less dice had it, the six temporary physicians Pyramid, Inc. subcontracted with to staff Cape Cod Community during its summer infusion of tourists were particularly good doctors, and the department, although extremely busy, ran smoothly. Pyramid, Inc., of course, had just fired shots in the dark. The pledge drivers, Norman's Kids, with their fingers crossed, had hired the first six doctors who responded to their advertisements for the summer casting.

But as dumb luck had it, there were no eight balls that year. In fact, the physicians were pretty much on the ball, and fortunately so, because it was a mildly disastrous summer with a large number of automobile-accident injuries, especially lower tibia-fibula "Volkswagen fractures," several near-drowning episodes, and a deluge of minor injuries, a veritable deluge.

Chief among these were the great number of hand injuries, especially the self-inflicted chain saw massacres the weekend woodsmen from Boston suffered. Mahoney could always hear that predictive sound on his way to work, "Bzzzzzzzzzz." Aristotle said, "The hand is second only to the eye." Although a little numbness on the lateral side of the index finger in a bricklayer might not be bothersome, the exact same deficit can ruin the scholarship chances in an aspiring pianist to the Julliard School. Classical anatomy refers to the "artist's and the artisan's" nerves of the hand. The diagnoses of some injuries to the sensory branches of the "artist's" nerves can be quite subtle, but the Hershey Medical Center was a good training ground, and Mahoney picked up three diagnostic coups, although the patients themselves never knew what good pickups they were. In fact, most of the time patients were unaware when they were receiving large-Cat care versus Monk medicine.

One woman was even greatly annoyed with Mahoney when he insisted she return to Boston for microsurgery of a severed digital nerve for what she thought was just a trivial puncture wound, but had she not had the surgery, she would have been plagued with a lifetime of numbness on the inside of her thumb. Still, her parting words to Mahoney were, "I only came in here for a damn tetanus shot."

Some nights the emergency room was so packed the waiting

time to see the doctor was over three hours. A camaraderie occasionally developed among the menagerie in the waiting room requiring crowd-control skills on the part of the nurses and doctors. One night the emergency room was so over-crowded, it functionally closed, and a group of exacerbated patients in the waiting room began to develop an identity all their own, creating a fearsome touch of anarchy in the air by midnight.

Also, during the months of July and August, the hospital held noon medical conferences devoted to speakers on medical, surgical, or pediatric emergency medicine topics. The talks were integrated with other medical conferences held in the area. Since the hospital served sandwiches at the noon conference, they were well attended by the doctors. In addition, the speakers and visiting physician audience got a tax deduction, being able to write off part of their vacation expenses for attending. These physician jamborees, with live, in-person lecturers, were a surprisingly rational use of the tax code, encouraging cross-fertilization from geographically diverse and outspoken groups of physicians, for when these physicians got together, they shop-talked of nothing but medicine.

Doctor **Hell**-on-Therapy Westerly summered on the Cape for several weeks each year, looking surprisingly lithe in a bathing suit. He was immensely entertaining, with a brand new repertoire of medical-toxicology stories which he loved to tell. Some of the side effects he described hadn't even appeared yet in the *Physicians' Desk Reference.*

In mid-August Adkins, Steinerman, and Dan Anderson visited the Mahoneys for several days. Adkins and Steinerman arrived first, everyone meeting at a local seafood restaurant. The restaurant was a favorite eatery of doctors attending conferences in the area. To everyone's horror, the insufferable Jonathan Stullman happened by on his way out and sat down. He certainly looked a little worn from his orthopedic residency, and told everyone how much he hated Johns Hopkins.

"You know how they pick the women students at Hopkins?

Their admissions committee chooses the ones least likely to interfere with the male's study habits."

Actually it was kind of funny, and everyone laughed, but they didn't extend any cordiality. Stullman said he was tired, excused himself, and they all breathed a sigh of relief.

As doctors do whenever they form a quorum, they became intensely engaged in a conversation on a medical condition. Tonight's topic; Lyme disease.

New England was an endemic area and the disease had recently become epidemic on Cape Cod where as many as twenty per cent of the ticks carried the spirochete (an infectious organism similar to bacteria and viruses.) Most of time the disease presented with a characteristic red rash in its first stages, and Mahoney said the Cape Cod Community Hospital was seeing about three cases a week.

At this point, a certain ritual had to be played out while the conversation went up a decibel. It always infuriates doctors who see patients to listen to pathologists and radiologists make suggestions, especially high-minded ones, on how clinical doctors should be evaluating patients. It makes the pathology and radiology crowd livid at even the merest suggestion that they should confine their opinions to things they know something about.

Adkins fired the first round that night. "You know what upsets me about you guys who are seeing these patients. I think every patient should be fully undressed and evaluated regardless of why they came in. I'll bet you'd pick up more erythema chronicum migrans (the bull's-eye, concentrically-ringed, red rash of Lyme disease, sometimes seen with the tick still attached to the patient at the center of the first ring). "I'll bet...," Adkins continued, but now watching out of the corners of both eyes as the Cats were getting ready to spring. "I'll bet you guys would pick up a melanoma every year just by examining every patient without their...," but it was too much for the Cats, Mahoney leaping first, unable to let Adkins finish.

"That's high-steppin' horseshit, Paul. You see yet again, you just don't how things work outside of your corner of the hospital, or is your office in the hospital anymore?"

Steinerman couldn't hold back any longer either. "That is such crap, Adkins, do you realize how many patients I see in a twelve hour shift? There's no way I can tell the nurses to 'fully expose' every sore throat or sprained ankle, every fish hook in the hand or foreign body in the eye, every splinter, every..."

But Adkins didn't come ill-prepared, quickly throwing some napalm on the fire while fanning the flames. "Those patients shouldn't even be coming to the emergency room anyway, Abe. Half the time they're there cause the hospital advertises so much, especially that ridiculous billboard on the edge of town with you guys on it," shouted Adkins, ruffled by the innuendo about not talking about things he didn't know anything about.

Mahoney and Steinerman were enraged by the statement it was their fault patients were over-utilizing the emergency room with trivial complaints, but Adkins stood his ground, "What about nurse practitioners or physician assistants? They're not being properly utilized either."

Now Tahoe's glandularity got pinched as she Virginia Woolfed with, "A doctor still has to see every patient, Paul. You should see these people around here. They demand everything, and they'll insist upon being seen by a doctor, even if it's just so they can act like an asshole."

"Look," continued Steinerman, "it's the physician right down there in the pit actually seeing the patient who's got all the responsibility. That's the captain of the ship for his or her twelve hours, not you Monday morning autopsy quarterbacks at Death and Doughnuts. The emergency physician is the one who's going to take it on the chin if Lyme disease is missed in its first stage."

"Yeah, but that's just what I'm saying, you guys wouldn't miss it if you just undressed every patient," Adkins continued on, getting louder and louder, making internists at nearby tables unable to finish their fresh, wild-blueberry pie.

Just as half the restaurant rose to go wilding on Adkins,

Dan Anderson finally arrived. Dan was in town for the New England conference of hospital administrators. He was now the administrator of a rapidly-growing hospital in southern New Hampshire, which had itself become a bedroom community for the growing city of Boston. His emergency department was staffed by a group of six dedicated emergency physicians who distributed their income equitably, democratically shared night, weekend, and holiday shifts, and were not "managed" by a "suit."

"You should see," Dan told the group, "the flood of glossies that arrive when the administrator has a stable group of E.R. docs. The crips and the bloods chomp at the bit trying to steal their contract and suck some cream off the top. But I'm a man of experience now," as everyone laughed, "and I throw the promise-laden glossies, full of daffy 'products' and 'services,' into the incinerator. I've got to tell you about the 'mosquitoes.' "

"Mosquitoes?" asked Tahoe.

"Well, you see," Anderson continued, "all the 'management' groups come to the hospital administrators' meetings, setting up elaborate booths in the exhibit area, full of their commission-driven marketing people known as contract-acquisition specialists, but which I nicknamed the 'mosquitoes.' One of their mosquitoes stays in the booth while the rest of the road show starts landing on the hospital administrators, and start stinging like mosquitoes.

"If you turned to the right, a mosquito approached, telling you the quality of their doctors and services. If you turned to the left, another aggressive mosquito would sting with the quality of their contract doctors."

Anderson told how he suddenly saw Bing. Bing was doubling that day as a "sidekick" and a "mosquito."

"Bing didn't recognize me, bumped into me head on, landed right on the tip of my nose, and stung me," while everyone roared with laughter, finally able to finish that pie.

"After first looking at my name tag, Bing began with, 'Our group, Mr. Anderson, is called Pyramid, and its founder, Doctor Norman Lyle,' " everyone chuckling again, "have the highest quality, board-prepared emergency physicians in the entire nation," making the jubilant audience laugh loudly. "'They are backed up by a professional management team with literally, Mr. Anderson, millions of hours of experience and the resources to make your emergency care team the highest quality in the nation,' " which made everybody howl.

"Quality, quality, quality," quipped Anderson, "the mosquitoes love to sting everyone with the word quality. They piss quality out their bladders and shit quality out their assholes. They're all fighting for a share of this extremely lucrative 'management' marketplace. It's the only specialty I know of spawning this perverse, brokered industry of middlemen who seem to make all the money, and with no one to regulate or stop them.

"By the way, the American Academy has a new president, this N. C. Kensington. Anybody know him?"

Adkins replied, "Yeah, I remember Kensington. The guy with the big cranium. Not really acromegalic looking, a normal physique, but a disproportionately large head. I don't know much about him, but he seems like a nice enough guy."

"Well, keep me posted if you hear anything. I just mailed him over fifty glossies instructing him to use them for fertilizer. I also told him to let me know if they find a vaccine for the Anderson Syndrome."

The Dan Anderson stories got funnier and funnier as he spoke of the outrageous shenanigans of the crips and the bloods trying to steal away the "management" contract from the six, independent, board-accredited physicians working in his hospital. His best story was the one about the conniving crip who, in desperation, finally showed up himself in the emergency room as a patient "with chest pain," trying to maneuver a letter of introduction to Anderson, offering him a Loch Ness Monster-Chardonnay lunch followed by tickets to the Boston Red Sox playoff games.

The next morning, breakfast was held at the Mahoney's on an open patio, served on a large, transparent, glass table. They sat on white, wrought-iron chairs, all of them wearing bathing suits. Toward the end of the brunch, while sipping his third Bloody Mary and slowly chewing on the celery stalk, Mahoney suddenly looked rather quizzical.

"What is it, Philip?" Steinerman asked.

"Paul," said Mahoney, "what did you mean last night when you said 'that billboard with you guys on it'?"

"That idiotic billboard over by the duck marsh next to the highway," replied Adkins.

"What's everyone talking about?" said Tahoe.

"The billboard, the billboard. You guys know what I mean," shouted Adkins.

Mahoney, Steinerman, and Anderson looked at each other as Tahoe repeated, "What are you talking about, Paul?"

So Adkins just stuffed them into the Jeep Cherokee he'd rented for the week, and drove the doubting Thomases out to the recently erected billboard on the outskirts of town, and when they got out of the car, they stood in perfect silence looking at the huge billboard advertising the Cape Cod Community Hospital's emergency room:

"staffed by Pyramid's Quality physicians"

It had twelve-foot-high cutout pictures of Mahoney and the five other doctors with their heads irregularly cut out on the top of the humongous billboard so the doctors looked like Mount Rushmore presiding over the Canadian Goose Marsh Preserve.

Mahoney gasped, looking at his four-foot-high, long thin face in a coronal plane, and heard Adkins say, "SEE!"

Gazing at the latest gimmick of emergency medicine "management" drummed up by one of the mosquitoes at Pyramid, Inc., it was Tahoe who first burst, and the five of them roared and roared and roared with laughter, falling to the ground.

Mahoney was finally able to speak, "It's from those pictures I had to smile at the birdie for at the beginning of the summer."

It was truly an unbelievable sight, and a perfect cap to Adkins' summer, tax-deductible visit.

The racketeers grossed a windfall that summer with Pyramid's six doctors working through the busy season. Lyle calculated after malpractice, supplies, and even the extra fifteen-thousand-dollar commission he gave to the mosquito, Tim O'Fallen, for snaring the kitchen scheduling contract away from Goldman to fill in the summer blanks, that he averaged a little over seventy-five dollars an hour clear profit, seventy-five dollars and fifty-two cents, twenty-four hours a day, seven days a week for the twelve weeks of summer on Cape Cod. Norman Lyle looked at that finger-lickin'-good check for $152,248.32, realizing something about gastroenterology that summer, learning there was a greater fortuna in emergency medicine "management" than there was in shit.

As for North Adams, Cro made sure, of course, Pyramid, Inc. was thrown out of the Berkshire Community Hospital after their one-year contract was up, giving Goldman the "management" contract the following year. Monk was thrown out of Holyoke six months later than everyone predicted, and since he'd never worked at North Adams and hadn't signed the sacred writ of the noncompete clause, he was picked up by Goldman and made the director, Monk's third emergency-room directorship in two years.

It was now early fall, and the turning of the leaves signaled Norman Lyle to embark again on one of his many European vacations, this year for two whole weeks in his beloved England. Lyle was most dangerous when he was in London, especially in the early evenings when he slowly sipped his favorite liqueur, Benedictine and Brandy, his B & B in the quietness of the "library" attached to their room in the "Bed and Breakfast" townhouse where he and the former Carolyn Skanks always stayed.

On his third night, while very relaxed, Lyle was thinking about a clip he'd seen on the television show *P.M. Magazine* concerning advertisements by supermarkets and their competitors using a "loss leader," an item marked down to below cost to attract customers into the store so they would buy other more profitable items as well. He was intrigued, pondering the concept of a loss leader. "A loss leader" began to stir in his mind, "a loss leader," how interesting.

Sipping the B & B liqueur, he also thought of all his contract hospitals, and how his crowning achievements had given him money and visibility. But Lyle knew he lacked something, something that his portfolio of sixty-five "management" contracts, many of which had come and gone, hadn't given him yet—a reference.

No clinical physician, no emergency-room nurse, and no administrator had anything good to say about the Pyramid, none Lyle realized. There was no one but himself or Bing to call for a reference. Suddenly the free associations synapsed. He reached out to call The Cambridge Clinic long distance, the primo diagnostic center in Boston, a very well-respected hospital.

Lyle got an appointment with the O-J-T-er of Cambridge Clinic, and getting that appointment was no easy task since the O-J-T-er was a savvy individual like Dan Anderson, remembering full well the fate of his old friend. He initially refused to have lunch with Lyle, but finally told him he could spare only twenty minutes. Lyle thanked the administrator and hung up.

Lyle realized how important it was to get a "loss leader," a hospital flagship that could be used in the future as a reference, and what could be a better showcase than The Cambridge Clinic? He would have to get it, and that's all there was to it, he would have to get the "management" contract, and personally "fill in the blanks" himself like a kitchen scheduler in hyperdrive. He would make the O-J-T-er an offer he couldn't refuse, then hire the best doctors, swallowing the monetary loss, and he would get a reference.

Pouring himself another princely aliquot of B & B, the unremitting ache arose within him again, that feeling of not belonging, the bitter resentment of his childhood as Lyle sat there still seething at Francis Peabody, even though he and Carolyn had just remodeled his old estate.

Lyle knew he needed more than a loss leader to assuage that destructive feeling that was about to ruin his trip to London, where he felt the most comfortable. He thought deeper and deeper, coming up with his second scheme that night.

He could endow a chair of emergency medicine in a great university, an endowed chair that would live on and on, and maybe, Lyle thought, getting drunker, maybe one of Peabody's great-grandkids could end up the Norman J. Lyle Professor of Emergency Medicine at Harvard or Stanford. He began to realize this would go hand in hand with the flagship hospital. Lyle knew organized emergency medicine had long since crossed the boundaries of any form of respectability, but these were two magnificent ways to get back his own respectability, using the pattern of the robber barons of old. With respectability he knew he would lose the ache, because men with respectability don't have a need to fit.

Slumbering in the oversized chair, Lyle thought of new flagships like the Naval Hospital at Annapolis or maybe the Mayo Clinic? Pretty soon he could have four or five selected references, removing the last road block to the growth of Pyramid, Inc.

Lyle chuckled, realizing it was all conceived in the great City of London by the shining light of Piccadilly, out of a simple supermarket ploy.

CHAPTER TEN

THE OTHER SIDE OF MIDNIGHT

"If you don't like the news, kill the messenger."
—*Ancient Greek saying*

N C. Kensington could be summed up in one phrase, he was a nice guy. He'd just been elected president of the American Academy of Emergency Physicians, a certainly honorable culmination of a fairly distinguished career, although not the career path he'd originally chosen.

He'd been through the Goldman-Lyle circuit, but only briefly, and it was unclear to everyone whether Kensington just ignored the scams or was simply slow to smell the coffee. He chose to follow the well-established dictum that the discipline of the unregulated "free" marketplace of organized emergency medicine would somehow wave its magic wand clearing up the whole mess.

It was time for Kensington to head downstairs to a breakfast meeting with the general membership of the Academy in the Plaza Hotel in Copley Square. The meeting was a so called "policy" meeting, and Kensington was serving his figurehead role today. The breakfast was served with Plaza quality silver and china, and plenty of service. As the juice glasses were being removed, the cereal was served, but N. C. Kensington couldn't eat the corn flakes. Ironically, it was the cereal that drew him into medicine in the first place, and its vitamin fortification that eventually ruined Kensingston's dream of becoming a burn surgeon.

When Kensington was a college junior, he got a summer job at the corn flakes plant sweeping floors. His father knew a cousin at the plant who got Kensington the job, one plum of a summer job in those days. Kensington was still somewhat uncertain of his future, albeit a very promising future for the very bright and talented athletic student.

One Friday afternoon, an employee, a middle-age, overweight woman, was walking along an unprotected catwalk from the corn flakes to the sugar frosted flakes side when she tripped on the iron grating and fell into an uncovered, three-hundred-gallon vat of sodium hydroxide. The alkalinity of the sodium hydroxide made it ten times more caustic than Drano and twenty times more so than Liquid Plummer.

Without a moment's hesitation, Kensington ran over and pulled the screaming woman out by the hand, chemically burning his own hand in the process which to this day has discolorations and scarring. Without a second's thought of his own danger, Kensington dragged her immediately and appropriately into the industrial shower, rinsing her of the sodium hydroxide solution under a continuous steady downpour of cold water. He screamed for help, and the Econolines were summoned.

After just a few minutes, the shower began to overflow and Kensington was standing ankle deep in chemically-burning water. He screamed at the men who'd gathered to "do something." One worker suddenly realized the drain was plugged up, causing the shower to overflow like a little waterfall.

The drain was indeed plugged up because so much of the chemically-burned woman's top layer of skin, the epidermis, had sloughed off of her. Sheets of her skin formed clumps which blocked the drain. A worker took a broom handle and pushed the clumps of denuded skin away from the drain opening, allowing the water to escape. Kensington held her up, continuing to shower her for a full fifteen minutes. She never lost consciousness as most burn patients without smoke inhalation usually stay wide awake throughout their ordeal. She made it to the Econoline and the burn unit where she spent seven brutal days suffering third degree burns covering eighty-four per cent of her total body surface area.

Kensington visited her twice while she was grafted virtually from head to toe with an experimental pigskin. He developed a friendship, an attachment to her. Two days after the accident, she seemed to be doing better as the high-dose penicillin analogues being given round the clock seemed to stem the tide of streptococci that were beginning to invade her vulnerable body, devoid of its protective skin covering.

On the fifth hospital day, she deteriorated, and while being turned for a dressing change, one of the nurses saw the innocent-appearing, but telltale raised bump on her left leg, a little bump, but as distinctive as one of Jenny's petechiae. When the sun's rays caught the bump obliquely, everyone could see its ever so slightly greenish tint. Suddenly the patient coughed, and the glistening, almost transparent, emerald-green sputum signaled the nurses it was over.

The greenish-pigmented bacterial organism called Pseudomonas *(Sue-do-mon-as)* was using her body as a petri dish to grow like a bread mold, and since the penicillin had killed off all the staph and strep, the bacteria had no competition. Opportunistic organisms became runaways, seeding themselves throughout her lungs, kidneys, liver, and skin using the bloodstream for transportation into every body cavity. The burn surgeons gave her a different class of antibiotic, a potent poison called gentamicin, and at first many of the tens of millions of bacterial organisms died, but somewhere in one of those body hollows, natural selection had its Darwinian way, and a mutant strain emerged, mothballing the antibiotic. In fact, the resistant, smarter, and meaner Pseudomonas bugs began eating the antibiotic gentamicin for lunch. She died on her seventh hospital day of overwhelming sepsis, and her death hit the sensitive Kensington very hard.

Subsequently, Kensington saw several employees splashed with hot sugar just before it was sprayed onto the frosted flakes. Most did very well, but he watched in amazement as some of their burns slowly evolved over the hours from a simple sunburn to a watery crop of blisters, a few of them later requiring plastic surgery. He studied how sugar at two hundred degrees would be expected to generate that type of burn. Both the caustic and thermal burns intrigued Kensington, like it had Lyle before him, and the surgery fascinated the brilliant young Kensington.

Kensington also attended the meetings of the federal Occupational Safety and Health Administration, OSHA, to evaluate employee safety. He saw how regulation was a necessary element in company safety to diminish the appreciable risk to workers, and how regulations had to be implemented by a government agency with some teeth to give the company a nudge to spend some greenbacks on non-income producing investments in employee health.

This accident happened, of course, in the days before OSHA became a real force to be reckoned with, the Henry Ford-like days before regulation. The young Kensington boy knew someone had to alter the worker's exposure to risk, especially when it involved simple actions costing so little and not detracting from commercial production. Certainly everyone at the corn flakes plant was grateful when OSHA put a lid on certain unsafe practices.

Kensington dreamed of the day he would become a burn surgeon running his own burn unit at a major university hospital, and perhaps discover a cure for the invasive bacterial infections in burn patients.

Even though the sodium hydroxide vat now had a cover on it, the cat walks were still without side rails, and on that fateful day in August, the promising Kensington boy tripped on the walkway, falling into the brewing vat of the sixteen essential vitamins added to the company's cereal products. Although Kensington couldn't swim, the slurry of biotin and

Vitamin E kept him somewhat afloat in the five thousand gallon stew of nutrients listed on the side of every cereal box. As he lay vertically head downward in the enormous vat, he thought of how stupid it was to trip on the walkway, laughing at the act until he lost consciousness.

A black worker, Mr. Grimes, saw Kensington's left foot sticking up from the vat, and immediately pulled him out while Kensington sputtered A and D from his clogged jowls. The Econolines were summoned for the second time that month, and he was rushed to the General where a prominent niacin flush was noted in the now babbling Kensington. He was diagnosed with mild, hypoxic brain damage from the oxygen starvation while submerged in the B complex, but one of the eccentric internist-nutritionist researchers at the General felt strongly that the damage was not due to lack of oxygen, but the acute overdosage of riboflavin. After falling into the sixteen essential vitamins, Kensington, although still quite intelligent, lost his single-minded ambition to become a burn surgeon. The acute insult also caused his head to grow, but no one knew why. It was just his cranium that enlarged, his brain staying the same size. He became a somewhat odd looking fellow,

After his rotating internship, he began to fill in the blanks for Lyle and Goldman, wandering from emergency room to emergency room. He served on several committees in the Academy, and began evangelically preaching unity between the "suits" and "scrubs," always rambling on about everyone's being "one happy family."

All this background laid the foundation to Kensington's becoming the new president of the American Academy of Emergency Physicians, his huge cranium giving him the outward appearance of a very bright individual, a great figurehead at the head of the table and in front of the cameras at Academy functions.

As members of the Academy receiving a free breakfast and a tax deduction, Mahoney and Steinerman were also in attendance at the Copley Hotel.

Kensington gave an upbeat state of the union address about his first year as the new president of the Academy. Lyle and Goldman were there as well listening to every word Kensington said, looking for any signs of tinkering within the Academy, but empty-vessel Kensington remained close-to-the-vest, babbling on about gun control, motorcycle helmets, fetal rights, and a few other irrelevant right-thinking causes, and then commented on "the history" of emergency medicine.

Even though legitimate emergency medicine was founded in the Detroit, Rocky Mountain, and Los Angeles areas, Kensington said a great deal of good old-fashioned Yankee ingenuity and independence was necessary to create this new specialty.

Goldman and Lyle nodded with approval. Nothing on the noncompete clauses or "management" was mentioned, nothing at which to raise their entrepreneurial eyebrows. In fact, Kensington said outright, "The Academy cannot dictate business matters. That's up to you guys." The "suits" knew they were going to like this tranquilized, large-headed president of the Academy, hoping they might be able to re-elect the stubborn Yankee again and again.

When the breakfast ended, Mahoney and Steinerman had to run for cover as many crips and bloods were approaching them to work in their newly-opened (minor) "emergency rooms." Steinerman asked Mahoney about them.

"Well, Abe, in addition to Kensington, It seems New England has made one other tangential contribution to the world of emergency medicine, the so-called 'doc in the box.'"

"Oh, yes, I've noticed those little blockhouses opening all over the affluent parts of town. I heard they started in Rhode Island. Who works in them?"

"They house a physician with an active, unrevoked, state medical license. For lack of a better term, these little clinics call themselves 'emergency rooms,' usually 'minor' emergency rooms. Although to be fair, some of the owner-occupied 'doc in the boxes' are quite good. It's the discount brands that are built, owned, and 'managed' by the 'suits,' and staffed by God knows whom." The smiling Mahoney said, "Conventional wisdom has it that taking a sick kid to a non-owner-occupied 'doc in the box' is a form of child abuse."

Steinerman laughed, "Where's Paul Revere when you need him?"

"Let's head down to the White Horse Tavern," Mahoney suggested, but Steinerman had to run home to take a nap. He was beginning a shift at five o'clock that afternoon at one of Pyramid's very busy suburban (major) emergency rooms.

Shortly after Steinerman arrived at work, a call came crackling over the radio from David Minors, one of the city's best known paramedics:

> Base station one, this is paramedic six-eight. We have a twenty-eight year old black male who is out of control, and is presently behaving in an extremely abusive way. We can't smell any alcohol on his breath, but this guy seems drunk or high on something. We were called by his neighbors because he was out in the yard aimlessly squirting his garden hose into the air and...
>
> Paramedic six-eight, this is base station. What are the vital signs (blood pressure, pulse, respirations, and temperature). Over.
>
> Base station this is paramedic six-eight. We don't have any yet. It's all we can do to keep him restrained. He's a spitter as well, so watch out when we arrive. Our ETA (estimated time of arrival) is three minutes. Over.
>
> Paramedic one, this is base station. We'll call the police and we'll be waiting. Over.

When the paramedic rig arrived, the staff saw the deliriously manic, burly, black man restrained as best as possible. He spit on the nurses and that's always a bad mistake. There's an illusion that goes around the lay community that it's the nurses who really care about the patient, but even if that were the truth, spit changes everything.

Proper medical protocol dictates all irrational, delirious patients, including spitters, along with convulsive-seizing patients, and unconscious patients, be assumed hypoglycemic until proven otherwise. A hypertonic glucose solution needs to be pushed intravenously in every delirious, convulsively-seizing, or unconscious patient, via protocol, without a formal diagnosis. The proper role of the clinician is to behave like an automaton, giving the solution with the theory being that true hypoglycemia has so many variegated presentations, it can't be clinically diagnosed even by the most experienced large Cats.

Steinerman ordered the solution while the nurses begged for sedatives, various punitive measures, and steel handcuffs, when suddenly, Mr. Haydn Briggs "woke up," asked where he was, and mentioned he was a diabetic. Everyone stood back, including the police, as if a miracle had occurred. Fifty milliliters of a fifty per cent solution of sugar, sweet like a Chinese desert, given intravenously, had cured Mr. Briggs of his disease, true hypoglycemia.

The nurses understood immediately, having seen this many times before, and wiped the spit off of themselves, grateful that Steinerman understood the limitations of medical judgment, and had followed protocol, and not his, or theirs, or the paramedic's clinical instincts. Mr. Briggs was temporarily psychotic because of a common metabolic derangement, and had been treated by a protocol before a fair amount of physical restraint, dangerous restraint to the patient, had been applied.

Everyone of course had the bias. A combative, young black man found in the middle of the local ghetto was drunk, obviously drunk or drug crazed, and not hypoglycemic. Another half hour of restraint and diagnostic procedures would have left him as permanently brain dead as Sunny von Bulow.

Bias sets in many times during an emergency department shift. One can see zombified teenagers after a heavy metal concert, patients in a full cardiac arrest, a comatose young man after a near-drowning episode, but all are assumed hypoglycemic regardless of the circumstances at the scene, regardless of the prejudice, regardless of how many times one has seen it before. The physician must never set aside medical protocol, for sometimes only protocol can save the patient from the limitations bias imposes.

Steinerman had a long night seeing many patients. As it got later, the patients got more difficult and the doctors on call got more hostile. Just after three a.m. a set of stragglers arrived.

Patients signing in after midnight are always somewhat suspect, and patients arriving at three a.m. must be viewed with extreme, as they say, prejudice. Normal, balanced people, not in any particular life crisis, are not up and about at three a.m.

A funny thing also happens to doctors sleeping at home at three a.m. The same thought goes through every specialist's and subspecialist's dreaming mind. All practicing physicians have a seventh inning stretch at 3 a.m. They awaken and turn over, and while turning, are quite apprehensive. If they are not on call, they complete the one-hundred-and-eighty-degree rotation, and immediately and gratefully return to the rapid eye movement (REM) stage of sleep. But if they are on call, the phone rings. If they're lucky, it's a nurse from one of the hospital floors calling about a sleeping pill or a laxative for an inpatient. If unlucky, the phone operator says, "Standby Doctor, for the emergency department physician" (a.k.a. "the goddamn ER doc.")

The pediatrician on the mandatory call list might have to respond to a deteriorating asthmatic, a patient he or she doesn't know. He or she asks, "Why don't the parents have their own pediatrician? Maybe the child's simply visiting? But maybe, like the last time, it's because the kid's mother is suing her old pediatrician?"

Why should the orthopedists be called at three a.m? Because somebody fell out of bed? Oh, no. It's because a heavily tattooed, heroin-taking, uninsured, drunken motorcyclist has shattered his tibia and fibula, is now dripping bone chips on the emergency room floor, and screeching obscenities at the police. Why was the neurosurgeon called at three a.m? For the same doubly-handcuffed patient.

Why was the internist called at three a.m? For an elderly woman who stopped taking her diuretic and anti-hypertensive meds to protest the way her daughters were treating her, and was now in severe congestive heart failure. She brings her suicide note with her, giving it to the nurses immediately on arrival with the internist mentioned in the note by name. Both daughters are present, have to work tomorrow, and have children at home asleep with their husbands in alcoholic stupors. They want some sort of an answer, a convenient, painless one, and they want it now so they can get back to bed, back to REM. They want their mother's private internist there. Now! They don't want to speak to the internist themselves, they want the emergency physician to speak to the internist, to take their side, and give him or her a piece of their mind.

All these physicians have to roll out of bed and come to the hospital for ungrateful patients they would soon grow to hate, ungrateful, non-paying, demanding patients who might sue them later, putting their names in the local newspapers—like Bing's—as an incompetent, uncaring profiteer.

But more than that, it was the thought, yes, it was the thought that permeated their minds on the drive in, the thought that could be resurrected at staff meetings, that one universal thought, the only thought that all specialists in all specialties agreed upon, that three a.m. phone call, and what to do about the news. It was so clear in all their minds...*kill the messenger.*

Steinerman finally got to bed at five a.m. He was exhausted, and began to think again of that uneasy feeling the local doctors had toward him, something quite unlike the attitude exhibited by the physicians who frequented the Steinerman household when he was growing up.

It was the reason Bing had so much trouble going back to his old hospitals. Bing had been a very busy gynecologist who referred a great number of cases to the general surgeons, but Bing no longer referred big, non-emergency cases.

Doctors in Boston used to speak to Bing with, "Thank you, Doctor Bing, and as usual, you've made quite a diagnosis."

But now, with Bing's calling at three a.m. from the emergency room, the same doctors replied, "What?"

Steinerman was awakened at six-thirty a.m. that same night to see a young woman, Mrs. "MTV," who presented with an explosive onset of left-sided, lower abdominal pain accompanied by vaginal bleeding. The pain was unrelieved by aspirin, Pepto-Bismol, Tylenol, and the Ben Gay she had her husband rub onto her belly. The only thing which seemed to ameliorate the pain was lying perfectly still on the stretcher with her legs bent at the knees.

Steinerman suspected a ruptured tubal pregnancy, gave her the necessary fluids, called Adler, her gynecologist, and was accompanying her over to get a sonogram when Bing walked in. Steinerman wondered what Bing was doing there since Monk was scheduled to relieve him. Bing in a moment of drowsiness mentioned he was called by one of the "green pins" late last night.

"A green pin," Steinerman wondered as he sat in radiology, "What the hell is a green pin?" He suddenly remembered one of the technopranksters in Lyle's war room who told Mahoney and him, "The techs are not allowed to talk to the hospitals with the green pins because Pyramid already holds the 'management' contracts there." He suddenly realized if they already held the kitchen scheduling contract, there would be only one reason for the hospital to call Pyramid, Inc.—for a complaint. Of course, the green-pin department was the complaint department in the Pyramid organization, loosely called their "quality assurance" program. Obviously, obviously, the hospital was complaining about Monk, and obviously, obviously, Bing was the damage-control expert, relief hitting so he could put out the brush fire, to start-them-up-set-them-up again.

After Steinerman and his patient came back from the x-ray department, Eileen Chen, the radiologist, came over with the sonogram. She pointed out a left, para-ovarian mass showing fetal-heart activity, the absence of an intrauterine pregnancy sac, and free, unvesseled blood lying in the cul-de-sac beneath the cervix. Doctor Chen wanted to know who the surgeon was so she could call the surgeon herself, Chen always wary of emergency-room physicians.

Suddenly Adler arrived in the emergency room, looked at the sonogram himself, and then an explosion occurred. Adler disagreed with Chen saying the adnexal mass next to the left ovary was a benign cyst, and Mrs. "MTV" could go home. Chen strongly disagreed, saying the sonogram showed a classic, ruptured ectopic pregnancy.

Adler, however, stood his ground in front of Steinerman, Bing, Mr. and Mrs. "MTV," and the nurse. The argument escalated, Chen protesting loudly, when Adler, with an air of finality, said, "End of discussion. She's my patient. I make the clinical decisions and she goes home. Period."

Doctor Eileen Chen suddenly whirled around, grabbed Mrs. "MTV" by both lapels, and shook her. "MTV" winced every time the wave of unvesseled blood in her belly hit the highly innervated peritoneal wall.

"Do you want to die?" screamed Doctor Chen. "Answer me! DO you want to die? Die today? You need an operation. You need an operation TODAY or you are going to die. TODAY!"

Steinerman had never seen anything like this before in his medical career. Eileen Chen's voice screeched as she shook the victim and her misplaced fetus with its foundering fallopian tube, literally throwing her against the back wall. Steinerman,

Bing, Adler, the nurse, and Mr. "MTV" actually heard the succussion splash of free, unvesseled blood splashing against the raw nerves of her retroperitoneum.

When Mr. "MTV" saw Mrs. "MTV" wince, he realized, for the first time since they were married, that she took care of the children. He sensed something was truly wrong. He looked for guidance to the overweight, black vocational nurse from the graveyard-shift working overtime to pay for her daughter's vocal lessons who simply said, "She needs an operation."

But there was the "effective communicator," Bing, standing there. Bing knew if he spoke up to Adler that Lyle and Pyramid, Inc. might lose the emergency medicine "management" contract, especially since Adler was the chief of staff and on the executive committee. Bing also had some other information.

Pyramid had just made a ten-thousand dollar contribution to the United Jewish Appeal credited to Adler's synagogue. Bing thought about the proprietary information for a minute, but decided to maintain propriety, propriety at all costs, and knew it would be most improper for a "sidekick" to interfere with the relationship of a private doctor and his patient, that centuries-old, sacred tradition, more sacred than even the noncompete clause. Bing knew he was vulnerable so he took the better part of valor.

Bing had once been a busy private practitioner, an active member of a medical staff, fully aware of how things worked in the hospital. He knew the medical staff and board of directors would drop Pyramid, Inc. and can the O-J-T-er before they'd tangle with this little radiology ninja.

"MTV"'s husband did the first competent thing in his unionized life, taking his wife immediately to Fowler, the name on the mandatory on call list.

Doctor David Fowler was a kind of early Bing, and hearing the incredible story, knew Chen was right, knew Chen was always right and Adler was always wrong on a sonogram reading, and went ahead, knowing he might end up in a lawsuit. "MTV" was operated on that afternoon, and her ruptured ectopic was removed along with her left fallopian tube and disintegrated ovary. She required four pints of blood during and after surgery. She could have really used two liters of a problemless, intravenous saline solution prior to surgery, a more timely operation, and no blood transfusions at all, had she listened to Doctor Chen and the black vocational nurse.

Although "MTV" had a stormy course, developing an unusual form of hepatitis from the blood transfusions, she was in the fifty per cent who survived. During her subsequent pregnancy she went back to Adler, rumor being that she and her girlfriends preferred Adler's choice of suitcoats to Fowler's.

Steinerman sat on the desk staring at Bing. Bing pretended not to notice because he didn't want any confrontation with Steinerman. Bing knew Steinerman's father, and had used Doctor Steinerman many times in consultation when Bing's pregnant patients had arthritis or lupus. But Steinerman leaned over, quietly whispering, the nurses straining their necks to hear.

"You woulda let her walk out of here."

Bing didn't answer.

Steinerman said, "Have to talk to corporate first?"

Bing looked up and glared, threw the paper on which he was writing into the wastebasket, and walked away without saying a word.

Driving home that night Steinerman felt an uneasy feeling in his stomach. His mind was abnormally focused on one topic. He couldn't eat dinner for want of an appetite. He went to bed but he couldn't sleep. He lay there with a not unpleasant sensation in the pit of his stomach. It was something he hadn't felt recently, but knew the feeling from a long time ago, that peculiar crossroad of agony and ecstasy as he thought of Chen's hair catching up with her face as she turned and threw Mrs. "MTV" against the wall. Steinerman was in love.

CHAPTER ELEVEN

A ONE WAY TICKET TO PALOOKAVILLE

"Success has always been a great liar."
—*Nietzsche*

Nine months to the day after their encounter in the "quiet room," Tahoe gave birth to a beautiful, chestnut-haired, turquoise-eyed baby girl.

The Mahoneys had just bought a house in Braintree where Goldman had offered Mahoney a job at Braintree Children's Hospital.

In spite of the Loch-Ness-Monster lunch, the administrator of Children's Hospital was in the process of throwing Pyramid, Inc. out of their emergency department because of its dismal track record in providing adequate doctors, especially any with competence or interest in children's diseases or injuries. The Mahoneys moved to Braintree six weeks before Pyramid, Inc. was scheduled to get the boot from the booty of the "management" contract at Children's, and Goldman was moving in.

Goldman personally called daily to warn Mahoney not to work for Pyramid, Inc. in any capacity, and particularly not to sign any noncompete clauses at this critical time.

Like any good billiard player, Goldman was thinking two moves ahead, realizing Lyle was also having problems with three nearby, non-flagship hospitals, and wanted to persuade Mahoney not to work at any of the Pyramid hospitals. He gave

Mahoney generous commuting expenses to work in one of his own "managed" hospitals ninety minutes away from their new home.

Goldman lived in Braintree himself, making Children's a real trophy for him. He wanted the approval of local physicians, especially at the local medical-society meetings. Other physicians always asked, "What is it exactly you do, David?" Goldman never could adequately explain how he lived in Braintree, but kitchen scheduled emergency rooms in West Virginia and Montana. He was tired of being classified in his own hometown.

Tahoe was suspicious of all these phone calls, not fully understanding why Philip had to wait six weeks to begin at Children's, especially since the hospital administrator had taken the Mahoneys out to dinner, complaining of the nightmarish doctors Children's was getting lately to staff the emergency room.

It's well known when "management" groups are losing a hospital contract, the lame ducks take the opportunity to flood the E.R. with their worst doctors.

"Why can't Philip just start now instead of hobo-ing to this hospital ninety minutes from home?" Tahoe wondered. She listened to this business of contracts and noncompete clauses, instinctively knowing something was awry in the new specialty. She took one phone call herself from Goldman, Goldman quite happy to get her on the line so he could stress the importance of Philip's not working for anyone else in the next few weeks, particularly of not corralling himself into a noncompete clause, ruining his chances of working in Braintree, for anyone, in the next two years.

Goldman knew very well young physicians believed in the brotherhood of doctors, even kitchen scheduling, non-physician M.D.s, and knew the graduating residents and fellows never took the Benedict Arnolds or their quicksand contracts seriously enough.

When the time came for Mahoney to sign the contract,

Brother Goldman was away, and Mahoney, like most doctors, was ready to sign it without reading it, but Tahoe lined through the two-year noncompete clause, writing in six months instead. The pledge driver in charge protested meekly, but Tahoe insisted. The pledge driver just wanted to make sure they could fill in the blanks with somebody reasonable for the upcoming ninety-day probation. The pledge driver never did mention this to Brother Goldman.

When they got home after signing the contract, Mahoney had a message on his answering machine from Delorenzo, and called him back that night since both were emergency medicine residents together at the Hershey Medical School. He never paled around with Joe, but found him a straightforward guy, although somewhat boring, always talking about medicine, emergency medicine.

Like most newly-graduated residents, Delorenzo was a purist who viewed emergency medicine with rose-colored glasses. After his residency, he set up an optimal system of hospital contracts, holding contracts with three major hospitals outside of Cincinnati, and had twenty-two physician members of the group rotating shifts based on a computer program devised by Delorenzo. The income of the group was evenly divided based upon the number of shifts each physician worked, with incentive payments for doing nights and weekends. Delorenzo took fifty-six thousand dollars a year for managing the three-hospital group, a paltry sum by the "suits' " standards, not enough gold to even fill a tooth.

The "suits" would have easily soaked the three hospitals for a minimum of six hundred thousand, and most likely a lot more, a mere five hundred and forty-four thousand dollars more than Delorenzo took.

If the "suits" got the contracts, running the whole shebang, this mere five-hundred-and-forty-four thousand dollars that went to the physicians seeing and treating the patients in the emergency rooms, would instead go for the "suits' " recreation and retirement programs, the building of plush offices on choice real estate, the printing of glossies, the placing of advertisements in the journals for cheaper doctors, the hiring of sidekicks, mosquitoes, pledge drivers, green pins, red pins, corporate lawyers, contract lawyers, accounting firms, mergers-and-acquisitions specialists, the building of war rooms, the purchase of mainframes and FAX machines, and the installation of the latest AT&T equipment.

Since Delorenzo paid his physicians fairly, he didn't require pledge drivers or the Unisys mainframes, and since he believed groups couldn't optimally manage more than three local hospitals, he didn't hire mosquitoes, mergers-and-acquisitions specialists or corporate-finance transactionists. His group became a progressive model for the nation, a model literally shunned by many members of the board of directors and the corporate officers of the American Academy of Emergency Physicians.

Delorenzo himself was exceptionally competent and very well liked and respected, having been elected chief of the entire medical staff at one of the hospitals. Doctor Delorenzo was "quality assured" not only by the public, but by the inside track of the medical staff who had a different set of standards than the public. He, like Steinerman, was the so called "doctor's doctor," like many of the Cincinnati doctors who worked with and for him.

One of the first things Delorenzo did was eliminate a number of various activities taking place in many emergency rooms throughout the country, namely, other specialists performing procedures or doing risky treatments in the emergency room. There were many reasons for Delorenzo to do this.

Gastroenterologists have to sedate patients before placing the flashlights up their colons, and it was no secret, the more they "snowed" the patient, the further they were able to thread their light up that lucrative highway. Afterwards, they'd return to their offices, leaving the dazed patients to wake up in the back of the emergency room.

The hematologist-oncologists *(hem-onc)* gave blood-component transfusions in the emergency room, tying up a bed or two every morning. The hem-onc crowd was a pretty responsible group, but the transfusions were risky, involving chronically-ill patients who were time bombs if the smallest thing went sour.

The radiologists would immediately—and conveniently—ship over a patient who had an allergic reaction to the iodine-based contrast dyes, abandoning them to scratch their hives in the emergency room until they could be seen by the emergency physician.

The interesting thing about doctors is they love company when there's trouble. But the gastroenterologist can't call the urologist over when an esophageal blood vessel pops.

If a violent reaction occurs during a blood transfusion, the hematologist can't very well call the orthopedist over to help him out.

To whom do they say, "Hey doc, could you help me out over here?"

Obviously, obviously.

Everyone knows the first rule of medicine while in the emergency room is never to carry the casket yourself. Always include the emergency physician as a pallbearer if at all possible. The emergency room was a service station for many medical specialties, more or less a convenience store, and actually, it was indeed a miracle they just didn't put the giftshop in the emergency room.

But Delorenzo put a stop to it in all three hospitals, pointing out the emergency physician was relieved of all legal responsibility for these patients if a true emergency hit the emergency department. One heart-attack victim arriving by Econoline, and all liability would set with the hospital for the "boarders" since the emergency physician's first duty lies with the acutely-ill individual presenting as an emergency-room patient.

Delorenzo told the O-J-T-ers this was 1992 and everybody, including twelve-membered juries, were more sophisticated, making the O-J-T-ers squirm, readily aware he was right

Delorenzo pointed out the nephrologists never set up dialysis in the emergency room. They had their own center, and, even in emergencies, had their own dialysis room within the hospital, never dialysing a patient in the emergency department.

Delorenzo explained, "Ambulatory-care centers and day-surgery facilities are the optimal locations for these activities, and if the hospital would buy into them, it would make economic sense, remove liability from the hospital, and actually represent a progressive step for everyone." Even Cro-Magnon would have agreed.

A second problem Delorenzo had was a single orthopedist who refused to come in at night regardless of how emergent the patient's condition was, and emergent to Delorenzo meant loss of limb as he was not one to cry wolf.

Delorenzo had actually hired Monk once, and Monk's casting abilities became legendary. The casts were huge because Monk used an inordinate amount of plaster, and Monk's patients always went out with a Popeye arm. One three-year old once fell to the floor after getting off the stretcher, the weight of the cast following the law of gravity, clunking the tot to the ground when she tried to stand up.

Monk was let go by Delorenzo after two shifts, and after the Monk episode, Delorenzo drew up guidelines that all new emergency physicians were to be proctored by an experienced member of the group before any final decisions on hiring were made.

Of the sixteen orthopedic surgeons in the area, only one was a chronic problem. The other fifteen orthopods were very responsible, always coming in for open fractures and severe orthopedic conditions. As the chief of staff, Delorenzo threw some weight around, clearing up a problem no one else wanted to deal with, and things progressed in the right direction with only a few ruffled feathers.

Two of the administrators bought it, but the third wasn't

progressive to begin with, and the O-J-T-er enjoyed reading the glossies the "suits" regularly sent him. The O-J-T-er noted Cincinnati had a good football team, and he also liked golf, Beluga, and Dom Perignon.

One day Delorenzo noticed a peculiar sight at Good Samaritan Hospital—it was Bing. What was Bing doing here all the way from Boston in one of the hospitals in Cincinnati? Next he saw Lyle, Valerie Longo, the chartsy-graphsy couple, the administrator, the recently-hired assistant administrator, and then the gastroenterologist followed by the "chronic" orthopedist. They were all wearing golfing outfits, laughing, discussing some of the finer luncheon spots in Cincinnati, and which restaurant had the best filet mignon with the recently harvested morel mushrooms along with other delectable victuals. They were also discussing Napa Valley Cabernets, and, yes, who might win the Super Bowl this year, and of course, Pyramid, Inc. would have tickets for the game on nothing less than the fifty yard line. The wine, the steak, the scarce morels, and the sports talk worked, and the "effective communicators" convinced the O-J-T-er of Delorenzo's perceived deficiencies, and Delorenzo's contract was not renewed.

Bing came in for six weeks along with several other "start-up-set-up" physicians, and they were followed by the Jack Kerouac genre of Monks and Walshes, many of the new birds of passage traveling on Bekins Van Lines, recently (re)moved from Braintree Children's.

The gastroenterologist was allowed back in the emergency room, the "chronic" orthopedist slept at night while Monk Popeyed the toddlers, blood was transfused, radiology had their old refuge back, and for all anyone knows, the gift shop may have been moved.

Oh, yes, and Pyramid would receive one hundred and ninety-two thousand smackers a year for "managing" their one new client hospital (malpractice was covered by the hospital).

Forty thousand went for ongoing expenses to generate new contracts, ten thousand for the commission of the mosquito who snared the contract, ten thousand for the landscaping of the new satellite building in Saint Louis along with an original print for its stylish lobby, five thousand to the sidekick Bing, and one hundred and twenty-seven thousand dollars went into the back pocket of the ill-fitting Norman Lyle.

Delorenzo called the American Academy of Emergency Physicians immediately, outraged by what had happened. He told them this particular hospital was an historic event, the first hospital in the history of the United States of America fully staffed by residency-trained, board-accredited emergency physicians. These were doctors who'd spent four intensive years in a formal residency-training program earning their wings, and it would be a travesty beyond belief if it were taken over by a crip or a blood.

But poor Delorenzo had those rose-colored glasses on again. Joseph had forgotten the marketplace, been nuked by the "suits," and for the first time, realized the American Academy was the soft dick that it was. Kensington's synaptic network couldn't quite grasp the problem, but warned Delorenzo, "The Academy can't dictate business matters," and transferred him to Goldman.

Goldman almost laughed out loud at Delorenzo, wanting to tell him, "Hey sonny, this is the real world. Grow up and learn the bitter facts of life."

Actually, Goldman was extremely upset because he was staring at three yellow pins on *his* war room map placed on Delorenzo's hospitals. After hanging up, Goldman started his carousel turning, and it was off to the races on full red alert. He immediately called his mosquitoes, savagely screaming at them to change those two yellow pins to red pins, putting his mosquitoes like dogs on the hunt for Delorenzo's other two hospitals. Goldman had a certain respect for that crafty Lyle and his sidekick Bing, and he'd give anything to get a tour of Lyle's command center.

Goldman thought, "Good Sam of Cincinnati, such a well-known hospital, in view of one of the finest emergency medicine training programs in the nation, a virtual flagship hospital, a real trophy to 'manage,' and a profitable enterprise to boot. What a Brinks job.

"How did Lyle's radar pick up that window of vulnerability at Delorenzo's hospital? Emergency medicine 'management' is getting so fucking complicated," he thought, "I'm just going to have to pay myself more money for all this 'management' and 'effective communication.' "

But Goldman wasn't too worried, for his reconnaissance team had just landed an incredible coup. They'd kidnapped one of Pyramid's high-ranking mosquitoes, giving the rival mosquito a fifteen-thousand-dollar bonus. Of course, Goldman had no talent scouts looking for fine doctors, and a performance bonus to hire high-caliber physicians was an action no "suit" would consider to get the finest "scrubs" in their client hospitals. They actually spoke of it as "unethical."

But the "suits" figured what the heck, it's the marketplace. One get's a Monk, a Steinerman, or whatever, the only important thing is to be the lucky duck who got the contract. And there were no federal regulations to harness them.*The American Academy would see to that.*

The defecting centurion from Pyramid's office was able to give Goldman invaluable information, windows of vulnerability of client hospitals, profit margins of Pyramid's contracts, demographics delineating high-welfare versus privately-insured, highly-renumerative patient-payer mixes, profiles along with the sports, religious, and dietary preferences of various O-J-T-ers, but above all, a current Rolodex of available "scrubs" in the region, especially the personnel pool of Monks and Walshes.

The "management" battle was on and heating up, and the ranking members of the Academy claimed it was the American public and their children receiving all the benefits from this highly competitive, unregulated marketplace. Only a few disgruntled "scrubs" found this was not so good, for only a few knew what was going on. *The American Academy would see to that.*

Rumor spread quickly the hunting season was open, and miraculously, Delorenzo survived the assault on his other two hospital contracts, for the dogfight that erupted when the street gangs heard of his loss to Pyramid was intense as Academy approved group after frenzied group sent their bloodhounds out to try to demolish everything Delorenzo had accomplished. They flooded the administrators' offices with a blitzkrieg of glossies replete with buzz words and outright lies all calculated to weaken Delorenzo's image. Yellow pins became red pins on everyone's war room maps, mosquitoes bit daily, and sleazeball sidekicks schmoozed their way to power lunches, five-star dinners, and play-off games.

Delorenzo learned the hard way that providing the best possible emergency medical care to a community was not an effective anti-takeover measure, but Mahoney recognized the vast import of this much more than Delorenzo. Delorenzo was distraught, capable only of licking his wounds at the moment.

Mahoney pondered this for days, seeing a possibly unwinnable war as Pyramid's ugly tentacle had reached even Delorenzo's hospital. Mahoney reflected on these backdoor deals, with non-physician M.D.s bypassing clinical physicians in high-stakes dealmaking, leading to unimaginable bloated profits in the (black)marketplace. Sometimes, in just hours, incredible forms of newly-realized wealth were being created out of nothing as hundreds of thousands of dollars were raised and exchanged with more commodities added to the expanding and increasingly complex kitchen scheduling marketplace.

Mahoney saw the probability that truly expert, democratically-run, small groups with equitable income distribution would go the way of the California Condor, and fair-playing physicians (98.6% of physicians are fair players) were fighting a holding action at best.

For what if the crips and the bloods were persistent enough year after year, and if the mosquitoes bit continuously, being rewarded with hefty up-front commissions every time they scored a new contract, and if the administrator kept getting those slick glossies in the mail every day, and if the O-J-T-er liked Dom Perignon and Beluga, and football, and if...

CHAPTER TWELVE

UTAH

"In Utah, a Jew is a gentile."
—*Maxwell Wintrobe, M.D.*

Some people fit and some don't. Beautiful Chinese women not only fit, but are fully miscible within American society, and can attend any social function with a member of any race, always fitting.

A beautiful black woman is still notably black at all-white parties, and some physicians not only have to modify their storytelling, but also feel compelled to speak of other black physicians they know who are extremely competent or nice. No one feels compelled to tell Chinese women of Chinese physicians who are competent, nice, or who were classmates, and it is only beautiful Asian women who can move freely within all strata of all subcultures, fitting without question.

Asian women within the Ivy League collegian system come from two distinct groups, children of physicists and chemists, and the offspring of the owners of laundries and restaurants. They don't distinguish themselves as such, both fitting perfectly well within the system and with each other. As a whole, the group lacks a class system, or for that matter, even a desire for one. Their only distinction, then, exists through a dichotomy of dress codes, one group creating an identity by wearing impeccably-tailored clothes, usually designer labeled, but whether Roberta de Camerino, "Liz," or homemade, the clothes are fashionable, fitting like a glove.

The second group chooses to express the most dangerous gene of the Chinese female community, the herd instinct for squalor, found only on the X chromosome, needing a complete pair for penetrance, and requiring a critical mass of phenotypes for full expression. But because Chinese women are fully miscible within society, they don't aggregate, thereby never reaching a critical density, and thus, the chain reaction doesn't run wild, creating the actual and truly feared China Syndrome. If one wishes to see this genetic predisposition toward group squalor fully expressed scientifically, it's only necessary to visit any Chinatown in any major city in America, Europe, or Asia—except Singapore where it's outlawed—and smell the aroma, look at the cluttered streets, listen to the decibel level, and imagine what a group of coeds could do to a sorority house at the University of Southern California.

This second group of women, drawn in equal numbers from the physicists and the dry cleaners, incompletely express their DNA strand with the well-known, loosely-fitting, black-on-black-on-black attire, a peculiar cultivation of the Viet Cong look.

Eileen Chen was born in the lush Imperial Valley of central California, and her father and grandfather were so-so, ill-fitting farmers who barely eked out a living on the cash crops of broccoli and cauliflower grown on their small, rocky farm just a block or two from real fertility. But the Chen's family fortune took a dramatic upward turn with the Japanese internment during World War II as all of Mr. Chen's contiguous farmers were Japanese, and the Yamashtas and Egis were taken away on a one-day notice. They had become what was known as a perceived threat and, in reality, a real threat to the easy wealth of their ne'er-do-well Caucasian farmers. It was these neighborly family farmers, who through the California Agricultural Societies, bullied J. Edgar Hoover and Franklin

Roosevelt into interning these Japanese farmers so their neighbors could steal the richest farm land in America. Adkins couldn't have imagined land as lush as the California Imperial Valley, land so fertile Maine farmers stopped growing blueberries, so that plump, California blues could be served in Boston restaurants. But rather than having the one-day fire sale that most of the Japanese farmers had, the Yamashtas and Egis left their farms in the care of Mr. Chen, and he carefully tended the farms until their release date.

Mr. Yamashta was a renowned and somewhat reclusive farmer who grew large, luscious cauliflower heads, so large and juicy, in fact, that one year the University of California's agricultural schools bought his crops for seed. They named the subsequent seed line the Yamashta Cauliflower, which every farmer on the west coast subsequently grew as California further outdistanced the Midwestern, New England, and New Jersey farmlands.

Mr. Yamashta would come over to Mr. Chen now and then to give him some advice, but to little avail, because the Chens simply didn't belong in farming. After the war, Mr. Chen gave Mr. Egi's land back (most farmers at the time kept the land they "borrowed"), but Mr. Yamashta and his wife never returned from the camps. He wrote to Mr. Chen twice, and in the second letter, after his wife died, the childless and broken Mr. Yamashta, shortly before his own death, left the farm in a handwritten note to Mr. Chen.

The Chens farmed the rich terrain with ease. Their asparagus yields were never as high as Mr. Yamashta's, and although there would certainly never be a Chen Cauliflower, the family lived quite comfortably. They raised a typical immigrant family, and cultivated the education of their children better than the vegetables or themselves, Eileen growing up with violin lessons, Chinese school, and all the accoutrements of a middle-class life.

Eileen knew from childhood she wanted to go to the University of California at Los Angeles, UCLA, and only after her undergraduate years did she decide to go to the more high-brow University of Southern California, USC, medical school.

The Gentlemen's Agreement had it only the brightest Asians made it to the big schools, especially the ones with the sweetest bite of the academic cherry, the professional schools. Brown undergraduate, Yale medical, and Harvard orthodontics made it clear long ago they weren't about to carry this meritocracy thing too far. Regardless of the Asian over-representation of high-school valedictorians, the schools had no intention of undergoing Vietnamization of their campuses, except for the theoretical-sciences buildings.

Although Eileen knew she wanted UCLA, she felt obliged to apply to Princeton, getting accepted, but even she knew from the scuttlebutt she was far too beautiful a woman to gain admission to the Johns Hopkins University so she didn't apply.

Eileen Chen played the china-doll routine to the hilt, particularly enjoying Harry's Bar, a great watering hole for all species in which the men were trolling for the prettiest gal in Los Angeles. She and her roommate, Lily Kuo, loved walking down the chute with their long, slender, beautiful bodies with free-flowing, silken hair, immediately registering with the amygdala of every male at the bar. The big teasers enjoyed the fuming jealousy of their female counterparts, stealing the show while sitting in the mirrored corner yacking like they really had something to say to one another. Ah yes, these members of the UCLA *Woman Warrior* crowd weren't exactly members of *The Joy Luck Club*. They were gorgeous cockteasers with the overwhelming asset of incomparable beauty, and as Uncle Will once said, "Beauty provoketh thieves sooner than gold," and thieves there were at Harry's, that seventy-thousand-year-old watering hole with all the predators waiting for the vulnerable moments of their prey, waiting for them to put their heads down to drink.

Doctor Chen breezed through medical school, and like every beautiful woman her own age, had only one consuming outside desire, to marry someone as pretty as herself, which she did in her first year of medical school. She married a most handsome and very wealthy mandarin from Taiwan—also named Chen—whose family was in banking, and had moved to America when he was twelve. The marriage went rather well until her husband brought home, without warning, his mother, father, and aunt, and announced according to custom, they would be living with the Chens from now on.

Eileen prided herself now and then on being somewhat Chinese, but this was carrying the tradition thing way too far, and from then on the marriage turned sour. Daily battles ensued with Eileen becoming less and less Chinese, and her husband taking on more of the characteristics of the last emperor of the Chen dynasty in America.

But a most fortunate thing happened to Eileen Chen in her fourth month of pregnancy with her daughter, Annie Thieu Yen Chen, fortunate for them, if not necessarily for him. Her ex was crushed one night when his convertible car tumbled into one of the Malibu canyons rolling over several times. His family had a twenty-four-carat trust fund for him along with a number of large life-insurance policies, and the Chen's family fortune took a dramatic upward turn for the second time in Eileen's life.

Most of her medical professors felt Doctor Chen should have gone into surgery for she had quick and intelligent deft hands, and more importantly, she thought three dimensionally. Her visual-spatial conceptualizations made her quicker and more accurate than her contemporaries who went into surgery. The orthopedists at USC often joked about her obvious skills, claiming it was the slant of her eyes allowing her to see around corners, and her small, but authoritative hands responsible for those tidy suture knots deep within the pediatric acetabulum.

Had Eileen Chen been a first-generation immigrant, she probably would have gone into surgery, but being third generation, opted instead for the less arduous radiology residency with fewer nights on call. In the field of radiology she found a niche, her mind perfectly adapted to reading films with a certain intuitive notion, and from the beginning she seemed to get more out of an x-ray film than many of her colleagues.

After residency training, she left California to do a post-graduate year in Boston to master the CAT scan, and study what was to become her true love, the magnetic resonance imager. And there was another reason for the move.

Her daughter Annie was now four years old, and Eileen wanted her to spend less time with her increasingly-possessive in-laws, especially her mother-in-law, who was insisting Annie call her "mommie" instead of grandma. At the age of three, Annie also stubbornly refused to speak any Chinese, further complicating the family situation, and at four, refused to use chopsticks.

After the one-year fellowship, Eileen stayed in Boston getting a job at the St. Joseph's hospital as a staff radiologist. She implored them to expand the use of the magnetic resonance imager, but the older radiologists felt they'd done enough already.

Through the years the radiologists had learned how to read x-ray films, utilize radioisotopes, shoot dyes into patients' arteries and veins, and then, the formidable CAT scan interpretations. They felt resonance imaging was for the younger crowd, perhaps even a bit of diagnostic overkill, and there was another reason.

The radiologists in Eileen's department owned rather than leased their equipment. They had invested a lot of money in the already-outdated General Electric image intensifiers, so they wanted to get as much use and billings out of them as they could. They also had two years to go on their seven-year depreciation schedule, and early retirement of the equipment would mean recapture taxes on their original investment, thus offering them a strong disincentive to retool at the present time. This meant St. Joe's would have to wait at least another year for their magnetic resonance machine.

In the meantime, a mobile imaging van came to the hospital on Tuesdays, creating artificial tie-ins to the hospital admissions schedule. Then again, the fired Dan Anderson was no longer the administrator of Saint Joseph's, and a lot of departments took advantage of the latitude of the gracious Sister Mary Helen Terrence, the new hospital administrator as organized emergency medicine was beginning to fuck up the entire health care ecosystem.

Ironically, after her internship in general surgery, Eileen Chen had taken a year off to work in emergency medicine, and after that year, definitely decided to become a radiologist. She summed up the once and forever present state of emergency medicine in Los Angeles with, "I got tired of taking their shit."

At the time, Lyle and Goldman had "management" contracts in L.A., and several weasels holding single contracts were taking home stratospheric sums of money by fleecing the young "scrubs." Southern California was a good place for the more swinish of the unregulated kitchen schedulers to salt away a cool after-tax million in just a few years, quickly freeing themselves from any further financial worry. Eileen had also seen many Monks and Walshes, and like many physicians who saw the charade called organized emergency medicine, she never acquired much respect for emergency physicians, especially the ones working for Pyramid, Inc.

Although Steinerman was tall, good looking, humorous, and somehow didn't seem to "fit" in emergency medicine, Eileen still held him suspect, keeping him at a slight distance so Steinerman could never get Chen cornered alone long enough to ask her out. Steinerman knew if he asked her out in front of others, she would perfunctorily say no.

But there were always the techs, other physicians, or nurses around every time Steinerman went over to "clarify" something on an x-ray film.

Actually, Steinerman might just as well have asked her out over the hospital public-paging system since hospital employees have their antennae up at all times, are usually quite accurate, love discovering in-house affairs, and knew exactly why Steinerman kept coming over to re-check his own readings of the wrist and ankle films of his patients, and then only when Doctor Chen was scheduled to read. The x-ray crew and the operating room nurses are the best sources of gossip, and x-ray had Steinerman spotted a mile away.

Of course, Steinerman wasn't the type who backed down, so he asked Chen out, and she said no.

Doctor Chen had the suspicion all Asian women have when asked out by Caucasian men, even the ladies who only go out with Caucasian men, since the Asian affliction of white males is well known to them, forcing all of the beautiful ones to get unlisted phone numbers along with a restraining order or two by the age of twenty-five. They're especially wary of men who only go out with Asian woman, and worst of all, the Chinese freaks, the men who know all the dates of the dynasties of China, and that the Ching was meaner than the Ming one, always discussing shit Eileen Chen and Lily Kuo neither knew nor cared to know about, since roots was never really high on their agenda.

Steinerman had pretty much used up his approaches, so he decided, in one of his clever moments, to use a little bit of good old reverse psychology. He went into radiology one day and said, "You're such a stereotype."

Eileen whirled around, and for a moment it looked like she might throw him up against the wall rupturing his spleen or force him to drink some radioactive iodine, but he smiled quickly enough, stammering the way he did in Lyle's war room, "Just, just joking."

Eileen gave him the slightest hint of a smile, saying only, "Watch it."

It was after he lay in wait for her in the parking lot that he was finally able to snare a date with her. She was not a low-maintenance woman from the beginning, but it was a wonderful time for them. Being more than just clinically sound, the chemistry between Steinerman and Eileen Chen was quite correct, and it did lead to a covalent bonding which they both hoped would further recombinate a superior dynastic line, which in time it did. But perhaps more than anything, their relationship brought back an ability they'd both lost, the ability to laugh, to laugh the way they used to, an ability to laugh with one another. They fit together.

Some people fit and some don't. Tinsgley Harrison belonged and so did Sir William Osler. Sir William founded the world's first residency-training program in internal medicine at the Johns Hopkins University, and he wrote the first comprehensive textbook of internal medicine, a landmark for its time, and his clinical description of Typhoid Fever has never been matched in the English language. Osler also wrote a book of epigrammatic reflections which were brilliant, funny, and used freely in Kensington's newsletters and editorials.

But let's not give Sir William too much credit. After all, he did miss the boat on a few things. For example, he didn't believe in heart attacks. Sir William was also a phylogeny-recapitulates-ontogeny white-supremacist Englishman, a small-minded, bigoted little shit who was anti-Semitic, anti-black, anti-liberal, and anti-a lot-of-things. He was a member of the former aristocracy who sent all their children to medical school, strongly believing only children of physicians should be allowed to attend medical school. He did not belong to the new world symphony of upward mobility and intellectualism for all, but to an old order whose function was to preserve. He would have strongly disapproved of the daughters of Chinese laundrymen becoming endocrinologists or the sons of Korean fruit vendors studying medicine at the Hopkins. Sir William would not have fit in at the Boston Latin School, but did belong at Hopkins, where he indeed prospered, and certainly would have won the Nobel Prize had Uncle Alfred discovered how to detonate gunpowder sooner.

Doctor Tinsley Harrison was born to the landed gentry in Alabama, living in a different era, a genteel era before the

CAT scan, when American aristocrats sent at least one of their children to medical school.

Tinsley Harrison was a rich tradition in himself, a gracious, softly-tailored, well-bejeweled charmer who idolized Francis Peabody, an old Harvard blue blood, who once wrote in the *Journal of the American Medical Association*, "The secret of caring for the patient is to care for the patient."

No one ever quite knew what it really meant, but it was clearly humanistic, high-minded, profound, and zenlike enough for medical students to vaguely ponder when high. It was also an expression with such a wonderful ring to it, and like marching to the beat of a different drummer, it was so very New England. Kensington loved the expression, using it in every other newsletter. The crips and the bloods misapplied it in their glossies, and "...caring for the patient" flowed like cheap wine at all medical meetings, with full professors of medicine feeling naked without it.

Tinsley Harrison decided one day that internal medicine lacked an excellent textbook, and made it known he intended to be the editor-in-chief of the definitive medical textbook of the twentieth century. The Boston medical community was somewhat shocked since, although Uncle Tinsley had a world-renowned bedside manner, outside of cardiology, he didn't really know *that much* medicine.

But Uncle Tinsley did realize medicine was becoming more subspecialized, and envisioned a textbook separated by both organ disease and symptom complex, a textbook written by a variety of authors, all the best in their respective fields. The planning was slow and meticulous, and in a moment of utter sobriety, Uncle Tinsley Harrison placed a pivotal phone call to the most brilliant physician of his day, the most knowledgeable clinician of his time, a young man who was creating a new subspeciality in internal medicine called hematology, the phenomenal Maxwell Wintrobe.

Max Wintrobe, at the time, was an instructor at the Johns Hopkins University School of Medicine. Uncle Max discovered if one placed a small amount of blood into a test tube, it took a certain amount of time to settle, to stratify, to form a sediment. The rate of sedimentation became a yardstick of the acuity of a patient's disease process, used daily by rheumatologists like Doctor Steinerman. But even after discovering the landmark Wintrobe Tube, Uncle Max remained an instructor at the Hopkins, not an assistant professor, not an associate professor, not a full professor, not a Distinguished professor, not an endowed professor, just an instructor.

And so Uncle Tinsley edited and Uncle Max wrote, and the result was beyond anyone's wildest. Wintrobe's sections on iron deficiency anemias read like the Psalms; they were beautiful and literate. And his descriptions of the blood in a test tube, and how fast it settled, were simple and yet so accurate.

Harrison's *Principles and Practice of Internal Medicine* took the world by tour de force burying Osler's book, along with Osler, and it buried Osler's successors who tried to resurrect Sir William with a substandard sequel. "Harrison's" was read in Kansas and San Francisco, and it was read from Saint Louis to Singapore. It was translated into Japanese, while becoming fluent common ground with physicians in Spain, Italy, and the Communist block. It was the Bible of internal medicine, the Old Testament being the first sections on symptom complexes, and the New Testament going into the kidney, lung, bone marrow, and most recently, the immune system. Unbelievably, every edition got better as Tinsley wrote less, recruiting more of the budding Wintrobes of the medical community. The book belonged. It fit.

Then Uncle Max went on to elucidate the coagulation system, but still remained an instructor at the Hopkins. Unlike the Stullman family, Uncle Max didn't fit at the Hopkins.

One day an unusual call came from the University of Utah Medical School in Salt Lake City asking Uncle Max to become a Distinguished Professor, not just a full-tenured professor, not an associate professor or an assistant professor, and not an instructor. So Uncle Max moved, and went from being the lowest man on the totem pole to the highest. When he left he took Louis Goodman with him, and Goodman went on to co-write the world's best-read pharmacology textbook, and was also made a full professor.

Uncles Max and Louis realized there were only two types of people in Utah, Mormons and non-Mormons, and no one bothered to differentiate the non-Mormons into subgroups. Although they didn't fit, it was by not fitting that they did fit, fitting into the group of undifferentiated non-Mormons, gentiles as the Mormons called them, and it was in Utah where Uncle Max became a gentile.

CHAPTER THIRTEEN

PINNACLE, INC.

"General Motors doesn't make cars, it makes money."
—an old saying in Detroit

It was time for Steinerman to buy a new car. For the past twelve years, he'd driven a jalopy that was so rusty one needed a tetanus shot just to sit in it.

Mahoney was going to meet him at the dealership, and had arrived early at "Bill's New and Used Cars." After being descended upon by a locust swarm of car salesmen, Mahoney said he was waiting for Mr. Peter Lynch. Steinerman was caught in traffic and was uncharacteristically late. Mahoney watched Timothy O'Fallen, one of the salesmen, charm his customers as a middle-age couple approached the new Chevrolet Celebrities.

"Hi, I'm Tim O'Fallen. I used to be with the Ford dealership down the street, but the quality just wasn't there."

"Oh, really!"

"That's right. I'm the type of guy who has to stand behind his products in order to sleep at night. That's why I quit Ford and came over here. This is one car right here," banging his hand on the Celebrity, "that I can truly stand behind, and today is Manager's Day, so I can give you the deal of a lifetime."

"How much?"

"Before we talk price, let me show you these incredible features. Then we'll test drive this baby. There's only one of these left. There's a guy comin' back in an hour with his wife to look at it. This one's hot; it'll be gone today."

"Really?"

"That's right. We can hardy keep 'em in stock. In fact, since we're both honest men, I might even need a deposit before the other guy calls back confirming his offer. You know, then we legally have to accept it. I can tell right away, your wife will turn heads in this one."

"Really?"

"Let me get the keys. Wait till you get behind the wheel, you'll..."

Mahoney watched the new and used car shenanigans for over an hour, thoroughly entertained by one salesman after another. O'Fallen still hadn't made a sale, and was leaning against the Celebrity smoking a cigarette when Steinerman arrived.

"Oh, hello, Doctor," said O'Fallen.

"Oh, hi Tim. How are you," Steinerman reaching out to shake O'Fallen's hand.

"Shopping for a car? I can get you a good deal." There was a second of silence as the boyish Timothy O'Fallen sheepishly smiled, lowering his voice saying, "I mean it, Doc."

"That's o.k., Tim. My father's got a pre-arranged deal with Mr. Lynch. Dad's used him for years. You look good, how are you?"

"Fine, Doc. Really well. Haven't been sick or had to see Doctor in over three years. The pharmacy keeps my penicillin renewal going and I take it every day. I really learned my lesson this last time."

"Doctor" was what everyone called Doctor Steinerman. They didn't call him Doctor Steinerman or say they were going to see "the Doctor." They went to see "Doctor," and that's how all of his patients in the south end of Boston referred to him.

Doctor had treated Timothy O'Fallen for rheumatic fever as

a child, and O'Fallen had several recurrences because he and his mother slacked off of the prophylactic penicillin Doctor Steinerman prescribed for him on a daily basis. Three years ago, O'Fallen developed an infection on one of his distorted heart valves (damaged from the rheumatic fever), and this valvular carditis almost cost him his life.

When O'Fallen went to the county clinic, the heart-valve infection was immediately ascribed to intravenous drug use, the most common cause of valvular infections in Boston. Since most young physicians don't see rheumatic fever anymore, his valve infection was assumed to be the more garden variety. Between O'Fallen's Navy-acquired skull-and-crossbones tattoo on his forearm and his heart murmur, the bias had it he was a doper.

O'Fallen's mother called Doctor, who had O'Fallen transferred to a hospital a few miles closer to Doctor Steinerman's office and the O'Fallen home.

"What are you doing now, Doc?" queried O'Fallen.

"I'm working in emergency medicine."

O'Fallen went pale. Mahoney and Steinerman thought he was going to faint so they slowly moved forward to pick him up if he collapsed.

"You're an E.R. doc, Doc?"

"Yes, Tim. Are you o.k?"

"Does Doctor know you're an E.R. doc, Doc?"

"Yes, Tim. Are you sure you're all right?"

"Yes, Doc, fine." O'Fallen thought he might be able to sell Steinerman a used car after all.

"This is Doctor Philip Mahoney, Tim."

"Oh, yes, Doctor Mahoney. I remember you. Nice to meet you in person."

Mahoney did remember the voice, but couldn't place the face. Rather embarrassed, Mahoney said, "I just can't place you, Tim."

"I used to work for Pyramid, Doctor Mahoney. I used to call you a lot when we had E.R.s to cover."

"O yes, of course, Tim O'Fallen from Pyramid. I remember getting all those messages and calling you back, and yes, of course, Tim. Well, it's a pleasure to finally meet you in person. So, Tim, you also sell used cars on the side?"

"No, Doctor Mahoney. I quit the Pyramid. It's kind of a factory, you know. Besides, I took one of their real burn-out positions. I worked for awhile tryin' to get new contracts for them to manage, but it was too much pressure tryin' to get those hospital administrators to pick Pyramid over the other vipers in the snake-pit. It was good experience, though, and the commissions were great. They've got some top-notch salesmen in that organization. I'm sure glad they don't all work here. Doctor Mahoney, I hear you finished your residency?"

"Yes, Tim. I finished a residency in the specialty of emergency medicine, and am full-time at Braintree Children's."

O'Fallen looked at two of his medical idols in astonishment, and started to develop some valvular dysfunction. Finally he blurted out, "But that's a Pyramid hospital!"

"Well actually, Tim, it's now a Goldman hospital," replied Mahoney with a slight pang of embarrassment.

"But why do you guys do E.R.? Don't you want to be doctors?"

Mahoney paused, but Steinerman quickly said, "Tim, I'm interested in Pyramid. Come out with us tonight and have a few beers."

"But, Doc," O'Fallen protested, "surely you don't want to work for Pyramid, too? Didn't you go to Harvard?"

"No, no, no, Tim. I don't want to work for them. I just want to know more about them. I want you to tell Philip and me about them and how they operate."

"Well, that's quite a story, Doc. Sure, I'd be happy to." The puzzled O'Fallen agreed to meet the large Cats later that evening.

O'Fallen moved on when all of a sudden another salesman came up to Mahoney, extending his hand.

"Hello, Doctor Mahoney, I'm Alexander Coy Patterson, Jr."

"Oh hi, Alex. Nice to see you. Abe, this is Alex. He also used to call me from Pyramid's office."

"Nice to see you, Doctor Steinerman. I used to call you, too. In fact, I met you the first day you came to Pyramid. But actually, Doctors, I didn't call you from Pyramid. I got a big bonus from Doctor Goldman. I called you from his New England regional office from the Rolodex I pinched from Pyramid." Alex gave them a broad grin.

It turned out four of the six smiling, used-car salesmen in Bill's New and Used Auto had worked in one capacity or another in Lyle's or Goldman's operations—or both.

The large Cats and O'Fallen teamed up later at the White Horse Tavern, Mahoney and Steinerman first checking to make sure Jonathan Stullman wasn't there.

O'Fallen had already arrived, and the loquacious O'Fallen began chatting, going nonstop through the first six Molson Ales.

"Doctor Mahoney and Doctor Steinerman, you guys shoulda been there in the good old days. We had this guy Doctor Walsh."

"Walsh? We know Walsh," said Steinerman.

"Really? Doctor Walsh is still around? I thought he lost his Massachusetts license. Is he still a lush?"

"He's been three sheets to the wind every time I've ever relieved him," replied Steinerman.

"Yeah, but good old Doctor Walsh. No matter how drunk he was, we could always bank on him if we could find him. One night we went over to Doctor Walsh's house to sober him up. I drove while Alex gave him coffee in the back seat. We had to take the flask away from him before he went into the emergency room, but the important thing was, we got the blank filled. Monday mornings Doctor Walsh would come to our office, still half-nailed, and we'd pay him his show up money so he could go get stewed again. Doctor Lyle was adamant, though, Doctor Walsh couldn't work in those states where his license was revoked. Doctor Lyle had us check that out to make sure he didn't work in those states. Doctor Lyle also had us buy those dependency videotapes for him as part of our quality assurance program."

"What about Monk?"

"Monk! You guys know Monk? Doctor Monk was our favorite pack mule. We tried to keep him workin' twenty-four hours a day, seven days a week. Monk was great. Poor guy, though. Half the time he didn't know what time zone he was in. We sure got a lotta mileage outta him, but he fucked up so much we had to keep movin' him. We used to call Monk the defective O-ring of medicine, but he's such a nice guy, always tryin' to help out whenever he could. Last I heard, he was out in Western Wyomin' still workin' for the Pyramid. Doctor Goldman's always tryin' to steal Monk."

"Tim, tell us more about the day-to-day operations at the Pyramid," prodded Steinerman, not wanting to get too bogged down in the personalities of Walsh and Monk, although Mahoney was still quite interested.

"Look, Docs, you gotta have gimmicks to stay in business, any business, but especially cars, and I guess, E.R.'s. For example, you gotta tell hospital administrators some tall tales, like you got all board-accredited docs waitin' in the wings. Everybody does.

"It's like this, I turn the odometer back on every used car that comes in. I gotta do it because everybody else does it. The customer knows we all do it, but he still wants to buy a car with sixty thousand and not a hundred thousand miles on it. If we get a new car repoed in the first week, we gotta zero down the meter to get a new car again. So it's the same thing with the hospital administrators. They all know we ain't got five board-accredited docs waitin' in our office to come into their backwater town, but they still gotta hear us say it. It's just part of the game.

"I'll give you another example. Last year the Feds cracked down on student-loan defaulters. They made it so the banks can't loan money to college boys who welshed, so Bill, the owner, started carryin' his own paper for these deadbeats. For a few extra points over prime, we'd get 'em drivin' outta the lot the same day. Sometimes we'd make it so we'd only back certain models that weren't movin'. If they gave us any lip, we'd politely tell those bandits they might be lookin' at some jail time for those government claims. If they squawked about how America's got no debtor's prison, we'd say, 'Well, look at the IRS. What happens to those guys who don't pay up?'" O'Fallen had to take a minute to laugh out loud.

"They come in lookin' for a Honda Accord, and we'd stick 'em with a great big old GM car with all the bells and whistles on it, somethin' those yuppies would rather die than be seen in." At this point all three of them were laughing. "It took the competition over a year to catch up to us, but we damned sure moved some inventory, great big Chevy's that otherwise woulda sat there on the lot till the year end rebates.

"Doctor Lyle's full of gimmicks, too. He coulda made the Edsel fly, and we'd still have explodin' Pintos if Doctor Lyle worked for Ford. It's all marketing and sales, and Doctor Lyle's a genius. He knows all the buzzwords the hospital administrators want to hear, and if we got shit doctors, then we'd offer the administrator some ridiculous horseshit calling it a 'product.' Doctor Lyle liked us to tell the boss men, the O-J-T-ers, that our physicians like to put on health fairs in community shopping malls, especially for the elderly. Those guys eat it up. Who the fuck knows why? Pardon my French, but who the fuck wants Doctor Walsh takin' their blood pressure or measuring their cholesterol in front of J.C. Penney on Sunday afternoon? But we tell the O-J-T-ers we put on these Senioramas and Phonathons," O'Fallen laughed, "and these are just a few of our 'products' the other 'management' groups don't have, and we'd get the emergency staffin' contract.

"We also used to give the nurses these little bullshit forms encouraging 'em to snitch on the doctors, and we'd call it part of the 'quality assurance' program. The nursing directors just ate it up like you wouldn't believe.

"In fact, Doc," O'Fallen paused a second and pointed at Steinerman, "I remember we got one about you for bein' too slow on some Spanish kid.

"Doctor Lyle can really bait the hook, playin' on the emotions of the hospital administrators, especially with all that torts and liability stuff. Then, if all the other party tricks were failin', he'd warn the administrators about patients choosin' other hospital emergency rooms over theirs. That really got 'em, even if their emergency rooms were swamped, ridiculously overcrowded. They couldn't stand the thought of patients going down the street to another hospital. Census was everything, and we had all kinds of visuals, especially our brightly-colored pie charts and graphs to show the board of directors of the hospitals. Then we'd take the O-J-T-er out to a knockout lunch spot and really pour it on. You guys oughta go and see one of Doctor Lyle's glittery, special-effects extravaganzas. It's a real show, let me tell you."

"We have," the large Cats softly answered.

O'Fallen sensed Mahoney and Steinerman were finding his stories a bit repellent, and he was beginning to feel a little like the messenger. He was annoyed the doctors were comparing him to Lyle.

"Hey, Docs, listen. I may sell a lemon or two, but I'm certainly not as unprincipled as the Pyramid. After all, you know, you guys are dealin' with doctors and peoples' lives, and, I mean, you guys just figure what the fuck, it's just the E.R. At least we make sure our cars have workin' brakes on 'em before we let 'em outta the lot, but old Pyramid ain't nothing but warm bodies fillin' in blanks, and they don't give a shit about who they send out for what job."

Mahoney and Steinerman, the "you guys," started squirming. "No one's casting aspersions, Tim, believe me," said Steinerman. "It's just that Philip and I find this fascinating."

"Yeah, you guys never get into any trouble, but at least once in a while, one of our guys gets nailed with odometer fraud. But listen, old Doctor Lyle has a tremendous jealousy of Goldman Enterprises, especially after Doctor Goldman bought those soda machines. Doctor Lyle was becomin' sensitive that Pyramid was somethin' of a joke in the industry, and he kept thinkin' of ways in which the Pyramid could be precocious."

O'Fallen spoke of how Lyle was also "getting a little weird," and had been reading Winston Churchill's writings, lecturing to everyone at Pyramid, Inc. in Churchillian tones, speaking constantly about how so many sick patients owed so much to the few who'd founded the specialty called emergency medicine.

O'Fallen then began a more frightening story of how "Winston" decided to go the route of respectability through more money-losing flagships, this time homing in on pediatrics.

"Doctor Lyle, after comin' back from one of his trips to England, called everybody in to announce a new company he was formin'. He called it Pinnacle, Inc., and Pinnacle, Inc., a division of Pyramid, Inc.," O'Fallen chuckled along, "was to be fully devoted to staffing pediatric emergency rooms."

Suddenly O'Fallen burst in uproarious laughter, "Of course, we had no pediatricians nor did we really have any interest in kids, but Docs, we were in the business of makin' money. Actually, we avoided the hospitals with large pediatric populations because Doctor Lyle knew a major fuckup in a big hospital could topple the Pinnacle early on. We picked midwestern states where Pyramid was less well known.

"We had mostly the usual junk-bond doctors, but were able to snare a few good academic pediatricians for a short time. It was simple to hire them since academic pediatricians also took the vow of poverty," O'Fallen chuckled. "Also, the pediatricians had no idea what we were up to.

"Our mosquitoes flooded the Children's Hospitals of the nation with flotillas of glossies, speaking of the QUALITY of our physicians devoted to serving children.

"But you know, Doctor Lyle's somethin' of a genius, a real trend-spotter, realizin' the eighties were a time of guilty parents focusin' on kids.

"Doctor Lyle loved new schemes. For instance, he'd always make us get the demographics of an area, and then we'd name a company like somethin' we thought the O-J-T-er would like to hear. Doctor Lyle made sure each hospital contract had a separate corporation with a different name.

"When we figured out what name the O-J-T-er really wanted to hear, we'd come in with that name. So some days we were Emergency Medical Group, Incorporated, and other days we'd be Emergency Surgical Group, Incorporated, and the whole thing got pretty creative. If there was a large percentage of trauma patients, we'd go in as Trauma Specialists, Incorporated.

"There was this guy in Illinois who vertically categorized the state's trauma centers according to the hospital's capabilities, and kept referring to various 'systems of care.' We named one of our companies Trauma Systems, Incorporated, and got a hospital near a big Pennsylvania highway intersection with a high trauma volume.

"Lots of company names grew out of our imaginative burst," O'Fallen continued, not able to contain his glee, periodically breaking out in a belly laugh, especially when he said, "and, of course, whether or not it was Pediatric Emergency Care, Incorporated; Trauma Specialists, Incorporated; Toxicology Specialists, Incorporated; or Emergency Surgical and Medical Care Specialists, Incorporated—you docs know the one thing all these companies had in common besides Doctor Lyle bein' a shareholder? It employed those two All-American toxicologists, traumatologists, medical, surgical, pediatric, and acute-care specialists. Yes, both Doctors Monk and Walsh, and they've both worked for every one of our fine cor..., cor..., corpoooooraaations," O'Fallen laughing so hard he couldn't continue.

As usual, the "you guys" were sitting there with their mouths open. After O'Fallen guzzled another Molson, he continued.

"Four times a year we'd go out to the Midwest tryin' to scare up new contracts. One summer I went wildcattin' with Alex, even though he was workin' for Goldman, and when we were drivin' by a maximum security prison, Alex said, 'Hey, look at that, would you?' We drove in, got to speak to the warden, and Alex said that Doctor Goldman was a specialist in managin' prison doctors, and we wanted to manage his prison health clinic. I couldn't believe it. It was a simple cold call, but within a month he got the contract for Doctor Goldman to staff the prison health clinic.

"You see docs, we got a commission of from five to twenty thousand dollars every time we got a set of blanks for the 'suits' to kitchen schedule, and an extra bonus if we could steal a 'management' contract from someone else.

"When we were at the prison, the warden asked Alex the name of his company, and I got a little scared thinkin' what the hell can we say? Gas Chamber Physicians, Incorporated?

"But Alex was brilliant, extemporaneously saying, 'We are called Correction Physician Specialists, Incorporated,' and the warden lit up. Alex continued with, 'Our group deals primarily with the medical and psychological problems of prisoners, and we give our doctors intensive training in security and other unique aspects of prison medical care.'

"We laughed so hard when we left the prison, sayin' Doctors Lyle and Goldman were no longer one-trick ponies.

"When we drove by a local college, Alex said, 'Let's do some more prospecting. Come on, you do this one.'

"So we drove in and saw the president of this college, and I told him I represented Student Health Care Specialists, Incorporated. I went on this big, long fabrication about our company and its interest in providing the best possible student health care doctors known to the medical world and, pretty soon, Doctor Lyle sent Doctor Bing in as our student health specialist. Then about a month later, we switcharooed Doctor Bing for Doctor Walsh, who was now also a specialist in correctional medicine and student health. Pretty smart guy that Doctor Walsh, huh?" as O'Fallen ripped, roaring again with unrestrained laughter, wiping the tears from his eyes.

Steinerman and Mahoney looked as wide-eyed and blank as Monk on the Death and Doughnut stool.

"It was real lucrative, but I just burned out of the whole bullshittin' thing. Don't get me wrong, though, we were successful beyond belief, Alex and me, real rainmakers for organized emergency medicine. In fact, Doctor Lyle used to send my wife and me to his condo in the Bahamas every year for bein' the top mosquito in the Pyramid.

"Still, I stayed with Pyramid longer than I wanted to because of the medical coverage. Since I got the rheumatic heart, most insurance companies said I had a preexisting condition, and wouldn't give me a medical policy.

"When I quit we were movin' in again on Ohio. Alex and I had an expense account, but we used to stay at this Steve Waterbury's house."

"In Cincinnati?" Mahoney said, suddenly sitting bolt upright.

"No, in Dayton. You guys know Waterbury, too? Steve Waterbury got thrown out of Good Sam in Cincinnati, which is where he went after Doctor Adkins got him thrown out of Dupage. Boy that Doctor Adkins sure gave Doctor Lyle some problems. He was one of the few who stayed a thorn in our side. You guys know that most staff doctors are too damn busy to give a shit who's in the emergency room, even if it's Monk fuckin' up.

"Old Waterbury's somethin' like Monk, and keeps gettin' kicked out of hospitals, but every time they throw him out he lands rightside up and calls us. He's a real pig, so we have to take him out to the best eatin' spots in town for a couple of weeks. Then old fatso starts diddlin' to undermine the contract of the docs runnin' the emergency room. Usually he can get 'em booted so he can give the 'management' contract to Pyramid, and stay on our Super Bowl guest list."

Mahoney and Steinerman's eyes were ready to pop out, listening to the excesses of the wrongdoers with their facile rhetoric. They looked at each other like twins simultaneously saying, "Delorenzo!" It was Waterbury that had undermined Delorenzo!

They were agog as Steinerman said, "Emergency medicine 'management,' the greatest hoax ever perpetrated on another group of physicians, let alone the American Public. Although it's very clever dishonesty, I guess it still doesn't violate the law."

"This is the marketplace, Abe?" said Mahoney with a chuckle.

Steinerman replied, "Only in emergency medicine, a specialty that's getting worthy of a 'Ripley's Believe It or Not' entry."

"Yes, but Doctor Lyle also found it very important to support the American Academy of Emergency Physicians," said O'Fallen, "he took all the phone calls himself."

Steinerman remarked, "Lyle did always ask me to serve on a committee or two with the Academy."

O'Fallen continued, "We also had to know the major players in the Academy and some of the prominent crips and bloods. Doctor Lyle made us scratch their names off of the mailin' lists of the glossies he sent around the country advertisin' Pyramid's and Pinnacle's 'services.' Doctor Lyle always said it was 'unethical,'" O'Fallen chuckled, "to advertise to the administrators of well run hospitals.'"

Steinerman said, "Aha. Of course, Lyle doesn't want to offend any of the major players in the Academy's inbred crowd. It's strictly the Delorenzos of the world he targets, insurgent groups of highly-trained physicians with democratic scheduling, profit sharing, and distribution of duties, but without the resources to defend themselves against the Oscar-winning marketing performances of the crips and the bloods. The Academy's got it's own nonproliferation treaty, sweetheart-dealing amongst themselves while the protectionist leadership sells out the general membership."

As O'Fallen continued giving the "you guys" the overview of

the sleazy underside of the lucrative world of used cars and E.R.s, Norman Lyle was on the other side of Boston typing a speech in his cozy turret in the left wing of the Francis Peabody Ponderosa. He'd finalized his donation for the endowment of the Norman J. Lyle Professorship of Emergency Medicine.

At first, a group of bloods had approached Lyle, urging him to join with them to endow a series of one-year fellowships, teaching emergency medicine residents literacy skills in "management." It appealed to Lyle at first, but then he realized that although there was nothing mysterious about the legerdemain of "management," short of a deathbed confession, the crips and the bloods would never let the new "fellows" see through the keyhole into the backrooms of the inner workings of the cartels.

When Lyle pondered the joint fellowship, he just didn't like the concept of "fellows" studying the Sphinx of "management" for a postgraduate year. Deep down he was also afraid other physicians in other specialties would laugh at him.

"A fellowship in 'management,' like gastroenterology, toxicology or cardiology? A fellowship in Pyramidology, Norman?"

Lyle was sick of being on the perimeter of real medicine, and didn't want to share his name with Goldman and the other crips on this new Rosetta stone they'd concocted. So he went ahead with his original plan to provide the sole endowment to a professorial chair in emergency medicine at a university medical school that, ironically, didn't even have a separate department of emergency medicine.

If this chair brought him sufficient acclaim, he would endow a Pyramid, Inc. Chair of Emergency Medicine at Stanford or UCLA. If the Pyramidology fellowships went well, he would just endow them with his own and Carolyn's names.

But now the time of recognition had finally come as Lyle walked through the college commons. Kensington, the large-headed president of the American Academy of Emergency Physicians, and many other high-ranking pretenders to the throne were there to share in Lyle's big day. Crip and blood luminaries came from all over the country, but many local emergency medicine specialists and professors were notably absent.

"Fuck 'em," Lyle thought, "the industry's real stars are here." He dined in the Revolutionary War room of the President's chambers, afterwards giving a noble speech about the changing role of the emergency department. The former-divinity-student's benediction was, as usual, magnificent, and his old rectors at Trinity Church would have been proud of him, watching the prelate Lyle read his epistle like Saint Paul to the Corinthians.

Lyle had learned a great deal from Valerie, and worked hard on his likability quotient, trying to catch up with Goldman's popularity. Lyle was now the honey-tongued champion of touchy-feely people skills. Any (insured) patient who arrived at the steps of an emergency facility was considered a true emergency, no matter how trivial their complaint was.

"After all," Lyle pontificated, "the patient didn't go four years to medical school to learn what illnesses require immediate care and which ones can wait till morning. That's our role."

Lyle then gave the obligatory, sixty-second segment of hyperbolic Rambo rhetoric on the designated villain, the evils of big government, ending with the requisite finale in his backcountry tone, "And like I always tell my physicians, in the words of that great physician and humanist, Doctor Francis Peabody," Lyle feeling the sweet revenge of his childhood on Peabody, 'The secret of caring for the patient is to care for the patient.' "

The "suits" smiled, loving it, noble principles and polite laughter.

There they were, the kitchen schedulers, a group of inveterate second raters with a colossal frat-house prank run wild, a junior-year abroad run amok, but embraced by the unknowing, and proclaimed as leadership by the self-anointed clerisy of emergency medicine. As Mark Twain said, "Prosperity is the best protector of principle," and these very prosperous men were now men of principle.

The "suits" loved the idea that "scrubs" saw patients while they made money, made money and lots of it, made money while they went to ceremonies honoring themselves, the American dream coming true for the ebullient "suits." Instead of con men they were now policymakers. Instead of the Lee Harvey Oswalds of the new specialty, they were the bold, innovative Lee Iacoccas, and instead of the real murderers of Jenny and Mary G., they were now public health officials. It was too unbelievable to be true. No wonder they fired Dan Anderson.

Lyle could see the recognition of the bluest of the old bloods, with their admiration for this combination physician, entrepreneur, and philanthropist. The ill-fitting Lyle had moved a few blocks east on Beacon Hill, and knew he'd be invited back for other ceremonies, pictures, and the respect his clever prosperity had bought. He realized Oscar Wilde was wrong when he said, "No man is rich enough to buy back his past," and even the "scrubs" working in the pit would curtsy to him now.

Although they were members of the Academy and had free tickets to the gala, Mahoney and Steinerman abstained. Instead, Eileen cooked Chinese food for everyone. After dinner, they decided to call Cecil Grimes, a black from the Latin and Harvard Med, now an internal medicine resident at the General. Ironically, Grimes had taken electives in the dead languages of both Latin and ancient Greek for four years, mentored by the few remaining dons unaxed by the Boston budget.

Cecil Grimes, Jr., whose father had pulled Kensington out of the sixteen-essential-vitamin vat, told them how everyone in the med school knew of Lyle and his autogenocidal company Pyramid, Inc. The medical students and residents had already created a contest to determine the "nickname" of the new chair of emergency medicine.

Grimes explained the ground rules of the new contest: the new title had to have at least three words beginning with the letter P—another triple P for medicine. Only a black with a tongue for Latinisms could have created these guidelines, and Cecil said appellations poured in all day from as far south as Jacksonville and as far west as Honolulu.

UCLA's program had the lead with David Bierman's affectionate entry, Pyramid's **P**ol **P**ot **P**rofessorship of Emergency Medicine. Bierman calculated Pyramid's "generics" placed in the killing fields of the nation's emergency rooms would catch up with Uncle Pol by the year two thousand and thirty. Tahoe and Eileen were on the floor with laughter as Grimes spoke over the speaker phone.

The Duke University's emergency medicine residency program had a virtual tie with Randy Peterson's Pyramid's **P**ontious **P**ilate **P**rofessorship, and the University of Chicago's Brian Accola's entry, the Emergency Medicine Chair of **P**iss **P**oor **P**hysicians.

Grimes was suddenly paged to the ICU and had to hang up quickly, but told Steinerman and Mahoney to call him back later in the week to learn of the successful winner of the many jingoisms this new chair of emergency medicine would generate.

CHAPTER FOURTEEN

THE MISSING CHAPTER

CHAPTER FIFTEEN

CHART WARS

"A well-known, unshaven, unkempt, foul-smelling, slightly-cyanotic, sixty-two-year-old alcoholic gentleman was carried into our emergency room by three million lice, all screaming, 'Please save our host.' "
—excerpt from the doctor's written note shown to the jury in a medical malpractice suit, circa 1977

In the old days, emergency department charts were somewhat abominable in their sparseness, physicians somewhat disinclined to make lengthy, hand-written notes about the patients they saw.

The Connie Thompsons of the world changed all that, making medical charts into legal briefs.

The medical chart for a one-centimeter, superficial laceration on the outside aspect of the small finger used to look something like this,

lac 1 cm.

When the charting became more "sophisticated," physicians became more verbose, and although the medical care didn't get any better, the record of the same care vastly improved.

When the smoke and mirrors malpractice crises hit, medical charts took on a Knute Rockne defensive posture, not that well-documented medical care wasn't a good idea, certainly long overdue, and, "If it wasn't documented, it wasn't done."

However, as with anything the "suits" did, it was overdone, and overdone for the wrong reasons. Now it was, the better and more detailed it was documented, the better and more detailed it was done. The "suits" gave themselves extra Krugerrands because they entered the new business of "quality assurance" and "risk management," seeing even fewer patients themselves because they had to spend more time telling the "scrubs" to write more on their charts.

The "suits" also noted that with the use of dictating machines, the "scrubs" would say twenty-five per cent more than if they had to handwrite it all. Sometimes the "scrubs" even grunted into seventy-five-thousand-dollar, computer-assisted, voice-recognition machines, cranking out even more verbiage, and generating laser-printed charts reading like textbooks. The kitchen schedulers congratulated themselves on this finding, giving themselves yet another raise.

Since they had to skim more money off of the fees of the "scrubs" to give themselves more money to work on "quality assurance," they had to hire less-qualified, lower-paid "scrubs" to see the patients in the emergency rooms. So the more time and money the "suits" spent on "quality assurance," the lower the quality they assured.

They also had to attend more meetings on "risk management," and the more money they spent on "risk management," the more they increased the actual risk to the sick and injured patients.

It also turned out, the more health fairs and other nutty "products" and "services" they merchandised to the O-J-T-ers, the less care they delivered to the "consumers of the health care dollar."

Pretty soon the emergency-medical charts became ridiculously elongated, and virtually impossible to do longhand. The same superficial laceration on the lateral aspect of the small finger required paragraph after paragraph of detailed medical histories, physical exams, descriptions of the suturing (some of the moonlighting residents also ordered x-rays of the finger and a blood test to determine if there was extensive blood loss), and the pain medications given. The computers also generated pages and pages of discharge instructions covering everything from persistent pain to the possibility of gas gangrene.

Eventually the superficial lacerations to the small fingers, which were successfully treated for generations with Band-Aids, were universally sutured, the cuts generating charts whose dictation took far longer than the suturing itself.

Since no one could scribble all this and function in a busy emergency room, physicians usually stayed an extra hour or two after their shifts ended to perform the acts of composition. But the ironies of ironies was indeed noted, because the charts worked.

If attorneys saw a detailed, neatly-typed medical chart with no boxes left unfilled, they were much less likely to file a nuisance lawsuit. Such a detailed chart indicated to the jury a concerned, meticulous physician.

If a lawsuit was not filed because of an extensive chart, it became known in medical-legal circles as a "chart win." If however, the chart appeared with only "lac 1 cm.," and a lawsuit was filed, it was a "chart loss."

Chart wars now rage in emergency medicine, and are viewed by the "suits" as a strategy to keep ripping off the "scrubs." They are the mainstay of what is called "quality assurance" and "risk management."

Incredibly, it was the prescient Monk who taught everyone this from his very first day in the emergency department, as scribe Monk always wrote irrelevant, novelette-sized charts on every patient he saw. Although he didn't know what they were or what they signified, his descriptions of petechiae rivaled Sir William Osler's. An astute law firm might see more than a few indictments in Monk's medical actions, but reality is still reality, and every one has been sued at least once except for Monk. Monk had seen, mis-evaluated, and checked-out many "talk and die" patients, discharging them to a premature Kingdom Come. Monk, the emergency medicine variant of the Boston Strangler, had also sent several children off to "go home and die" preventable deaths with his thumbprints on their neck, but it did not go unnoticed that General George Patton Monk never lost a chart war.

One evening, Steinerman relieved the well-documented Monk, and, as usual, the Generalissimo had a logjam of patients in the waiting room. The kitchen schedulers were well aware of Monk's snail's pace, the O-J-T-ers complaining that many patients left the emergency room without being seen because the wait was so long.

When Steinerman entered the hospital, he was taken aback by the sight of one of those soda machines, a huge, neon Pepsi machine shaped like a big fat can of Pepsi with it's convex belly sticking out into the waiting room. Slowly walking by it, Steinerman remembered Tim O'Fallen's mentioning Goldman and the soda machines, but he and Mahoney hadn't called Tim back.

Steinerman stopped, starring at the huge electroluminescent machine. Suddenly he jumped when the whole machine shaped like a big can started blinking on and off. He ran into the emergency room as the grateful nursing staff said right in front of the imperturbable Monk, "Thank God you're here. There's a sick kid who's been waiting for over four hours, and we think he's getting worse."

The sick boy was John Fay who had a six-hour history of abdominal pain and vomiting (a two-hour history of vomiting when he first arrived), and now appeared rather ill with exquisite, right-lower-quadrant abdominal tenderness in a stomach without any bowel sounds of activity. He was clinically dehydrated with dry, hot skin, sunken eyes, parched mucous membranes inside his mouth, and didn't produce tears when he cried. His attentive parents bought him several sodas from the Pepsi machine trying to get John to drink, which he did, and shouldn't have, since one prefers to take a patient to surgery on an empty stomach.

Steinerman ordered a blood test and urinalysis, gave the boy some intravenous fluids, and called the surgeon who wanted to know the results of the blood test before driving in on a Sunday afternoon, but Steinerman insisted Fay clearly had a surgical abdomen. The grumbling surgeon drove in, thinking all the while of how he was going to skin this insistent messenger if he was wrong, but the surgeon did know Steinerman was usually right, so he had asked that the surgical nursing crew and the anesthesiologist, Doctor Larry Capaci, be called in for emergency surgery.

Things went well as John Fay was wheeled into surgery. He was rehydrated, pain-medicated, and perked up quite a bit. When Capaci went to put the breathing tube into his trachea, the sphincter at the lower end of the esophagus—a circular muscle acting like a valve holding the stomach contents in place—suddenly relaxed. A Yellowstone Geyser of Pepsi Cola suddenly gushed up his esophagus under carbonated force, flooding his airway.

Capaci scrambled to find the trachea trying to place the breathing tube to secure the airway, but there was too much foam, and the suction machine gave out, as it always does in emergencies. Before the nurses could start the backup machine, the soda pop flooded the right-middle lobe of Fay's lung, and even with subsequent tube securement and drainage, the Fay boy went on to develop a pneumonia, a peculiar pneumonia where organisms don't require oxygen to grow. Resistant organisms emerged, the bacteria proliferated exuberantly, and within a week the Fay boy succumbed. It was a rough time for the Fays, and in time they sued.

The following day, Steinerman received a frantic call from "Weasel." "Weasel," as everyone called him, although never to his face, was the emergency-room director, and sole holder of the "management" contract at the Berkshire Community Hospital in the now very ritzy Western Massachusetts foothills.

Weasel was a natural outgrowth of the frenetic growth of

emergency medicine contract development. Weasel was of that species known as the "weasels," a species of the genus "suits," a virulent subspecies, far from endangered, and a rapidly-proliferating form of miscreants in the world of emergency medical care.

Weasel didn't consider himself greedy, wanting just one pie for himself, one whole pie, that is. He'd offered two fellow emergency physicians partnership status with full profit-sharing after two years, but when the two years was up, Weasel decided to keep the whole enchilada for himself, getting rid of the two "partners."

He utilized the chart wars to his own advantage, and when many, well-trained specialists started moving into the affluent Western Massachusetts region, he utilized the chart wars, and the so-called spit, shit, hip, and piss wars in a masterful coup to profit mightily in an emergency department seeing a well-insured, investment-grade patient population.

He did this by being there first, sucking up to Cro-Magnon (still on the emergency department committee, somewhat weary after throwing Goldman out after throwing Pyramid out), and by belonging to the correct synagogue (Cro's synagogue), and not just any synagogue, but the correct one.

Weasel took only day shifts, never working nights or weekends, rarely seen about the hospital on the other side of midnight unless he couldn't find someone to fill in a blank. This gave him several strategic advantages. First of all, he referred patients to daytime colleagues bypassing the on-call list.

When Cro received all his stomach and colon bleeds during banker's hours instead of on the other side of midnight, he was a happy camper. Also, Cro received the fee for flashlighting the patient rather than losing the fortuna in shit to one of the other gastroenterologists who'd recently set up practices in the area.

Weasel carefully worded the chart ("...and the patient specifically requests by name, Doctor [Cro]...") so that he could use chart wars in defense of Cro in case the other gastroenterologists started a shit war with Cro. The same went for the selected urologist from the correct synagogue receiving obstructed bladders in some very desperate, fidgety men (piss wars), and the orthopedist, quite grateful to win a daytime broken-hip (war) in an osteoporotic Medicare gal. In return, Weasel was allowed to suck the cream off the top of other physicians' fees.

"The messenger" also took on a different role in the daytime, sending pre-screened, insured patients (the so called "wallet biopsy").

Spit wars were uncommon, simply a peacock show of feathers, since most of the pulmonologists were too overburden to be bothered.

As for the primary care doctors, they remained uninvolved, and in fact, might as well have been from a different planet, too incredibly busy, swamped with patient care, care of the patient's family, E.R. calls, committee meetings, keeping up to date, dealing with insurance companies and the continuous stream of threatening letters from the medical records department.

The phenomenal financial success of the careerist "managers" went unchallenged, in part, because the kitchen scheduling fee of the relaxed "suits" was kept top secret, especially from the primary care doctors.

Weasel ensconced himself by forming a daytime misalliance with the heavy-hitting players performing pricey, big-ticket procedures—the cardiologist, gastroenterologist, orthopedic surgeon, and urologist from the correct temple—and was able to achieve the status of the referring general practitioner.

Weasel skimmed a cool, seventeen thousand dollars a month after expenses for kitchen scheduling one emergency room along with the false pretense of "quality assuring" and "risk managing" the single emergency room—not seventeen hundred, but seventeen thousand dollars a month after expenses for "managing" one hospital—and Weasel received cases of wine and scotch over the holidays to boot.

The night-time shifts and weekends were covered by the other two "future partners," local moonlighting residents, and a few of the young, recently-graduated, residency-trained, emergency physicians.

These grabby non-nocturnal weasels also saw the value of an institution like the American Academy, many of them quite active in it. It was no secret there were many weasels sucking in seventeen grand a month for kitchen scheduling one emergency room. They made it known they would drop out of the Academy, refusing to pay the dues money of the residents who worked for them if the Academy ever questioned their modus operandi. Kensington was well aware of this no man's land in his homilies, always referring to everyone in emergency medicine as one big happy family, with some of its members being quite a bit more well-rested, wealthier, and happier than the others.

Steinerman was unaware when he got that first call from Weasel that Weasel was desperate to fill in the blanks because he was getting rid of the two "partners."

Although it was a ninety-minute drive, Weasel offered Steinerman a good deal, so Steinerman decided to try it part-time, especially since Weasel said, "In two years, if you stay, I'll make you a full and equal profit-sharing partner."

Steinerman made his first minor sellout, agreeing to refer daytime patients requiring costly procedures to the local mafia. Weasel asked Steinerman to work many shifts because Weasel realized, like so many of his ilk, that he lost money every day he was in the emergency room actually seeing and treating patients. Patient care had to be turned into a sideline while he was out and about wheeler-dealering, particularly finding appropriate "scrubs" to see the patients, and then shortchanging them by taking his handsome cut out of their fees.

When Weasel became more active in his extracurricular activities, he gave Steinerman his day shifts more often. He rapidly became completely uninterested in seeing patients at all, something quite common with the "suits."

Weasel also decided to become more active in the American Academy, and at one of the Academy's meetings, Weasel stumbled onto another rain of gold. He was offered three hundred dollars an hour to review malpractice claims for plaintiffs' attorneys, and several thousand dollars a day to appear as an expert witness against other emergency physicians. He accepted, providing the cases and courtrooms were west of the Mississippi or south of the Mason-Dixon line so that no physician in his own medical community would know what he was up to in his spare time.

Weasel needed to become active in the Academy to offer a credential to the jury by saying, "Yes, I'm the chairman of the education committee of the Massachusetts State Chapter of the American Academy of Emergency Physicians, and that is why I feel qualified to testify in this case. Since I am also the director of a very prestigious Western Massachusetts hospital, and am on the clinical faculty of an equally famous medical school, I feel further qualified to testify in this case." It was just another racket which the leadership of the American Academy indulged in heavily, part of their cannibalistic philosophy growing out of the increasingly lucrative world of "quality assurance" and "risk management."

And, there was another reason.

Weasel hosted the subregional-chapter socials of the Academy, held at the "in" Sushi spot. He used these meetings to ingratiate himself with the new doctors, especially young residents, offering them an opportunity to become a "future partner." The only prerequisite was to do two years of night and weekend shifts, a little trial period to assure their quality.

The job went well for Steinerman, driving to the Berkshire Community Hospital three days a week. He and Eileen talked about moving there since Saint Joseph's still hadn't invested in a magnetic resonance imager, but Steinerman's small sellout was more than he bargained for.

Cro remained distant, asking only once about "Doctor," but

he offered no problems, and Cro had become rather skilled with the flashlight, and rather subselective in whom he scoped.

The urologist and orthopedist were both nice guys, very competent, and he got along quite well with them, but there was the cardiologist, and that was Steinerman's undoing.

The cardiologist, nicknamed ECHO, did an eight-hundred-dollar echocardiogram on every single patient admitted to his service, certainly a very safe noninvasive procedure, but even if ECHO's patients were transferred to a higher level of care within two hours of admission, the patient got the eight hundred dollar echocardiogram—and was billed for it—just before being transferred. Even if a ninety-six year old patient was within two hours of obvious death after admission, Doctor ECHO ordered the echo with the emergency echocardiogram obtained, and billed for, before the demise. ECHO felt, "Where there's a beat, there's a buck." ECHO had arm twisted his buddies into making him the only one allowed to read the eight-hundred-dollar echocardiograms, and he battled for this exclusive minion, even though there was a superlative cardiology group in the area.

The superlative group never asked the emergency physician about a patient's insurance status, always coming in to see new patients on the other side of midnight. ECHO rarely came in on the other side of midnight, especially important in these days of thrombolytic therapy for heart-attack patients. There was no ethnic rivalry since the superlative cardiology group was all Jewish.

However, they did belong to the incorrect synagogue. ECHO also got the superlative cardiology group barred from reading the electrocardiograms, having that chore farmed out to his internists buddies from the correct synagogue, who were not cardiologists. So the endocrine and gastro crowd did the official cardiogram readings for the hospital, which was not an excessive chunk of change in their pockets, but was easy work, keeping their kids in pocket money.

Steinerman referred his first set of chest pains to ECHO, but after the fifth patient he couldn't do it any more, so he began referring chest pains, especially in men in their mid-forties, to the superlative boys from the incorrect synagogue, getting away with it for some time using the chart wars technique.

But it couldn't work forever, and finally Weasel confronted Steinerman, telling him all cardiacs had to be referred to ECHO during the day.

Steinerman mentioned he referred all his stomach bleeds, prostate obstructions, and fractured hips to the boys from the correct synagogue, but just couldn't, in good conscience, send patients to ECHO because he felt ECHO, even though from the correct synagogue, was such an inferior cardiologist to the superlative boys from the incorrect synagogue.

Weasel hit the roof, reading Steinerman the riot act, and Steinerman agreed to do what he could, but it turned out he couldn't. Steinerman was caught red handed when he slipped into the hospital administrator's office one day, telling her the hospital needed a rotating, mandatory, cardiology on-call list for the protection of patients coming to the emergency room.

However, the O-J-T-er and her husband were members of the correct synagogue, and knew Weasel contributed twenty-five thousand dollars annually, so Steinerman was canned.

CHAPTER SIXTEEN

PHYSICIANS OF A LESSER GOD

"The phony exists in every vocation and has been vividly caricatured. Yet that which is comically ridiculous in other professions appears tragic when enacted by the physician. For he, more than any other man, finds his customers (the patient) completely at his mercy—they having placed themselves so deliberately. And when he distorts the facts of a case for his own rather than the patient's gain, he violates his exclusive position of trust."
—Oscar Creech, Jr. M.D., 1957

Mahoney called Steinerman, and with a near frantic voice told him to come to the White Horse Tavern.

When Steinerman got there, Mahoney was bubbling over with excitement, literally grabbing at him.

"Goldman owns the Pepsi Machine."

"What?"

"That's why he's being sued."

"What? Philip, what are you talking about? He owns what Pepsi machine?"

"Goldman owns the Pepsi machine in the emergency room and that's why he's being sued. Isn't this great?"

"What Pepsi Machine?"

"The one John Fay got the soda from."

"But that's Pyramid's contract, and I'm the one who saw the Fay boy after Monk bottlenecked everything for over six hours.

You're saying Goldman's being sued because he owns the Pepsi machine. What the heck...?"

"That's right. By the way, Monk's chart looked so good, he's not being sued, just you, Capaci, Pyramid, the hospital, and Goldman. The story is that Goldman got tired of all those law and business classes, going instead into the hospital concessionaire business. That's what Tim O'Fallen was trying to tell us when he mentioned Goldman'd bought those soda machines."

Steinerman was stunned.

"Look, Abe, Goldman's no fool. He did the survey, found out what the proletariat really wanted—or perceived they wanted—from their emergency rooms. So he put his enterprising mind to work to provide 'services' for the 'consumers of the health care dollar.' For sure he wanted to be on top of this one, and not let Lyle scoop him the way he did with Pinnacle, Inc.

"Rumor has it that Goldman got a good price on the machines since the prior owner was sued because the machines weren't properly bolted to the floor. Several kids in the waiting rooms started tipping them over, crushing themselves, and had to be sent to trauma centers."

Steinerman stared while Mahoney continued on about Goldman's new company, Hospital Concessionaires of America, Inc., with its growing number of franchises to put soda machines (and emergency doctors) into the nation's emergency rooms, but the big red, white, and blue neon Pepsi machine filled his mind like a new symbol, a perfect symbol for all of organized emergency medicine.

Mahoney said, "They're such big, beautiful, pearlescent machines, all lit up like that. Maybe Goldman could make them revolve? Or continuously blink on and off with an opalescent red, white, and blue? They're just so American as well, and maybe even a constitutional amendment against bashing them?"

Steinerman stared at Mahoney, and suddenly without warning, burst out laughing.

Mahoney tried to continue, but Steinerman convulsed with a bout of unrestrained belly laughter while the brilliantly-lit Pepsi machine took over his mind, demonizing him as he began to laugh uncontrollably, so uncontrollably he started to lose control of his voluntary musculature, his head hitting the table. Not inspiring any air for over fifty seconds, he couldn't speak, but Mahoney pursued his line of thought.

Steinerman started to beg the normally humane Mahoney, "Philip, puhlleeeeeeease..."

But Mahoney just said, "I think juke boxes will be next. Pyramid will place them in the waiting rooms. Then cigarette machines and video games will be Goldman's comeback."

"Philllaap staaaap," Steinerman cried trying to lift his head, only to have it clunk back down on the heavy wooden table, his ribs and abdominal muscles aching like a marathon runner, his entire body wracked with continued convulsive movements. His inspirations every minute or so sounded like a child with the whooping cough as he entered a dangerously anaerobic state, now becoming aware of his bladder, beginning to lose control of his autonomic nervous system as well, but the merciless, residency-trained Mahoney persisted.

"Pretty soon those crowd pleasers will invade the intensive care units. There're always families up there. There'll be no limit, a cappuccino bar in the radiology waiting room, a small French bistro for the doctor's lounge, and valet parking, of course. Possibly Lotto tickets could be sold, along with money-order sales and check-cashing services, all for the 'purchasers of health care.' If fact, what about a dynamite, live banjo band on Tuesday evenings?"

"AAAAUGH! PHILIP, FOR GOD'S SAKE I CAN'T BREATHE," Steinerman quickly said after a deep inspiration, his head banging back into the table while he began to fall off his chair, the phosphorescent can of Pepsi reducing him to a sobbing, quivering, helpless mass, the can blinking on and off, on and off, on and off taking control of his synaptic network. Suddenly, the huge Pepsi Can started to revolve around his cerebellum.

"You're right, Abe, the can should blink on and off as it revolves in the waiting room, on and off in the emergency departments, especially the children's hospitals staffed by Pinnacle, Inc."

Steinerman lay there, now having lost all control of himself.

"We could call it, 'Pinnacle's Hospital and Grill' staffed by Lyle's Good & Plenty physicians. The kids could be picked up by Goldman's 'U-maul-'em, we-haul-'em' ambulance service. The thumbs up their asses could mount the huge Pepsi can on top of the Sears Tower."

"AAAAUUUUGHHH."

"It could be four stories high, or even higher, like the billboard on Cape Cod, symbolizing emergency medicine and where it's going. The brilliantly-colored can could shine on the dark, windy Chicago nights illuminating Lake Michigan, a beacon to all wayward physicians in search of a blank to fill."

Steinerman was growing weak. "Ahhaaaaaaaaaaaaa...," now making frequent shallow gasps for air. Only with Mahoney's and several other patrons' help were they able to leave the White Horse Tavern.

When he got home, Steinerman tried to explain the Pepsi machine to Eileen, but she simply stared in disbelief, listening intently, worried it might be early meningitis.

But Eileen wasn't an emergency department physician, and the Pepsi can revolving on top of the Sears Tower could only make sense to an emergency "scrub."

Steinerman passed out, waking up around noon with a splitting bifrontal headache. Eileen had left an aspirin tablet and some Maalox next to the bed.

Trying to get up, Steinerman started laughing again, quickly grabbing the front of his painful, seemingly swollen cranium. He agreed with Mahoney. The can should only be lit at night and stay lit, stay lit on top of the Sears Tower, the brilliantly-colored can shining in the dark on windy Chicago nights, a "Bekin" to all physicians in search of a blank to fill for a pledge driver working for a kitchen scheduler. He chuckled again, watching the revolving ceiling fan begin to spin faster, even though they didn't own a ceiling fan, and he slumped back to sleep. Eileen had to wake him up when she got home at five, still laughing.

The Fay family's attorneys were also having trouble with the Pepsi machine, especially when it became a Subchapter S corporation with passthrough tax implications somehow entwined with the specialty called emergency medicine. The Fays' attorney called the American Academy of Emergency Physicians, but Kensington's brain trust was befuddled by the dizzying, partnership-passthrough concept.

"After all," he thought, "it couldn't save the O-J-T-er who died at lunch in 'the region,' " and so Kensington deferred to his own legal staff to make sense of this.

But it was one of Goldman's corporations, Hospital Concessionaires of America, Inc., which owned the Pepsi machine being sued in the John Fay case. Via some Lend-Lease Act, the emergency medicine "management" contract of the Braintree Children's Hospital was a wholly-owned subsidiary of which the sole shareholder turned out to be the Pepsi machine, holding as its single asset the noncompete clauses of the "scrubs" working there, and the "scrubs" were insured by a malpractice firm incorporated and headquartered in the Grand Bahamian Islands, which in turn was also partially owned by Hospital Concessionaires of America, Inc., and actually insured some of Pyramid's and Pinnacle's "managed" hospitals, as well, in some sort of legally acceptable reciprocal arrangement.

So, the "management" contract of Braintree Children's, which seemed to own the Pepsi Machine, was actually owned by this one busy Pepsi Machine, physically bolted to the waiting-room floor of a different hospital, but owning Mahoney's noncompete clause in Braintree, even though Mahoney was insured under a malpractice policy issued in the Grand Bahamian Islands which was partially owned by Hospital Concessionaires of America, Inc.

The headquarters of Grand Bahamian Island Medical Malpractice Corporation was physically located in a small office between an offshore banking firm, a South American drug dealer, and a well-known arms smuggler.

One could hardly fault Kensington for not having the intellectual horsepower to comprehend organized emergency medicine in anno Domini 1992.

But what about the liability? Who breached their duty to the patient, and was the proximate cause of damages? John was the sixth of eight children spawned by the Fay family so rapidly they resembled a litter, and his death was a sort of remedy unto itself for the Fays, but damages had to be assessed. Although the Fays were not the von Trapps, the family lawyers saw a set of electives in Greek and Latin, even though John was white, at the Boston Latin School, providing the state still had some money. They extrapolated a future in neurosurgery for John Fay, and so they had to go after the deepest of pockets.

The now tightly-bolted Pepsi Machine seemed to be owned by an endless set of abstractions, culminating in the bewildering concept of a Caribbean Island-insured emergency medicine contract at the Braintree Children's Hospital, holding Philip Mahoney's highly-restrictive noncompete clause as its single biggest asset. Since the maze had to involve the Mafia, Iran, Bolsheviks, and the Colombian Cartel, and had links to the Kennedy assassination, the plaintiffs conceded it was the wisest thing to go after the anesthesiologist. So they soaked Capaci's insurer for 1.2 million bucks, and Capaci never knew, and still doesn't to this day know, what hit him.

A few days later Mahoney called to remind Steinerman it was time to go to the American Academy's annual meeting, this year being held in New Orleans.

After a bumpy flight, they first entered the rotunda where the exhibits were displayed. A group of carnival barkers hawked and grabbed at Steinerman and Mahoney, pulling them into every booth they walked by. They had to chuckle, remembering Dan Anderson's stories, as they found themselves repeatedly stung time and time again, this time by the pledge drivers.

A pledge driver cornered Steinerman with, "and unlike other contract emergency medicine 'management' groups, Doctor Steinerman (a 'scrub'), ours is a QUALITY group with mostly board-prepared emergency physicians who believe in fair compensation (the 60/40 split), who want equity partners (the extremely limited partnership), who have the experience of a well-trained management team (the crips and the bloods), marketing services (the mosquitoes), and recruitment specialists (pledge drivers), and we (the 'suits') follow closely the guidelines of the American Academy of Emergency Physicians (the thumbs up their asses)."

Steinerman saw Mahoney who told him Pyramid, Inc. was offering a New Orleans bauble, the kind they throw from the floats at the parade, a thousand dollar "reward" (award?) for any doctor who found another doctor to work in their group for a year. Mahoney wanted to sign Steinerman up under him to get the door prize, both laughing at the finder's fee, the latest tactic in the recruitment of "quality" for the Rolodex. They finally made it outside at eight o'clock, noting a sea of backslapping "suits" milling around.

It was the annual awards dinner of the American Academy. The thumbs up their asses gave out numerous awards, usually to the crip or blood who had stolen the most money from the "scrubs" that year, and after lionizing one or two of the "suits" like they'd discovered the polio vaccine, they incidentally gave out a few research awards. Steinerman liked the research, and was the only one anyone knew who actually read the articles in the Journal of Rabbit Brain Death, the nickname for the Academy's monthly journal. He was rather impressed with the emergency medicine medical-investigation crowd, so he insisted they go to the hootenanny.

And what a Mardi Gras it was! The suits were all seated together on the "floats" in the front; a jazz band played while an incredible buffet of wine, Creole and blackened Cajun cookin' was decoratively presented. The "suits" buzzed each other with niceties, and Valerie Longo was so ecstatic Lyle had to spray the Pyramid float.

The mosquitoes were standing on their floats continuing to throw handfuls of brightly colored baubles at the O-J-T-ers. Maybe New Orleans would win the Super Bowl this year? The researchers were scattered about the room, not clearly identifiable. The female emergency physicians were surprisingly attractive and sleek, especially for woman physicians, and were distinguished from the "suits" as, for unknown reasons, there were no female crips, bloods or weasels, no entrepreneuses, just stylish female clinicians.

The pledge drivers ate and drank like condemned men, along with Mahoney and Steinerman. Suddenly it became wonderfully noisy, and in the mad excitement, Kensington grabbed the microphone, and started wildly throwing cherry pies at everyone—seat belts, air bags, motorcycle helmets, fetal rights, gun control, and child abuse, especially of the sexual nature. The "suits" sat smugly in perfect approval while the impetuous Kensington went on to give his usual ludicrous speech, only this time making it incredibly inane for the big fete. He spoke tearfully of the nostalgia (another form of lying) of their pioneering days, comparing everyone present to Neil Armstrong and the first group to land a man on the moon, not realizing the emergency medicine spacecraft had veered off course, landing on the dark side.

Steinerman and Mahoney loosened up, half-listening to Kensington's foolishness, pigging out with the pledge drivers, and beginning to feel a little weightless themselves. While the spread of wine and Cajun cooking continued, Steinerman thought maybe the "suits" and thumbs up their asses should present Death and Doughnut conferences—especially since there were less and less invitees attending D & D.

The next morning, the two darkly bespeckled "students" met at the "Hand" lecture. They listened to the humorous and informative orthopedist. Steinerman thought what a wonderful thing for an orthopedist to take several days off from his lucrative practice to teach the common and most serious errors made with regard to hand injuries seen in the emergency room.

It also occurred to Steinerman, it was a lecture of negative self-interest since the hand surgeon was giving them advice so he wouldn't get referrals. Steinerman was decidedly impressed.

The orthopedist talked about the examination of tendons in the hand, telling everyone to stress the tendons to see if they were partially cut rather than completely cut, to stress the tendons to see if they were just hanging by a thread.

"When you stress a partially lacerated tendon, ladies and gentlemen, and it suddenly pops, making a loud snapping sound, you have saved the patient a delayed diagnoses, so,

"never say OOPS, always say THERE!"

What a perfect piece of advice for any physician Steinerman thought. He would have to pass it on to Eileen,

"never say OOPS, always say THERE!"

The room ripped with laughter while the orthopedist kept repeating his advice. Everyone who saw patients had at one time or another found themselves saying "OOPS," but should have said for everyone concerned, "THERE."

The orthopedist continued, "Also, you all know the incredible resourcefulness of children to remove dressings, bandages, and casts no matter how carefully they're applied. Every morning you see a child who has removed the treatment applied the night before. Therefore,

"the smaller the child, the larger the cast,"

which made the physicians roar again, every physician knowing the average American preschooler is a Houdini. Of course, the cast had to be within reason, not a gravity-defying Monk

Popeye arm.

At the next lecture, a radiologist focused on "things not to miss," and her talk was excellent. How important it was to know how to read cervical spine films at two a.m. What good did it do for the radiologist to read them the next morning, six hours later (you "ain't" getting the radiologist out of his or her canopied bed from under those Laura Ashley sheets, and that's taken for granted in the community hospital). What does a physician do? Tell the now-paralyzed quadriplegic, "Oh, your x-rays were positive last night? Sorry I sent you home"—the "go home and get paralyzed" patient.

The ophthalmologists in their lectures also demonstrated what a minefield the emergency department was. Miss something down there at three a.m. and, well, the vision is lost. No second chances, no appeals, Doc.

In fact, let the wrong thing set for a few hours, and one would be consulting with the least desirable specialist, namely Adkins, and Steinerman noted there were no pathology lectures given by the medical examiners. The pathologist's job didn't begin until the emergency physician's task ended.

Steinerman went to the neurology session, nine hours total, spread over three days, and it was the finest neurology session to which he'd been, even considering the General's lectures. It was during the neurology lectures that Steinerman began to recognize the subtle changes that had taken place in his medical thinking during the past several years.

Headache? He used to think migraine and tension, but now it was brain hemorrhage, meningitis, and abscess. Weakness? He used to think chronic disease, multiple sclerosis, thyroid, but now it was botulism, acute brain dysfunction or myasthenia gravis. His thinking had changed from the internal medicine checklist to the emergency medicine checklist, which were the same diseases, but the list was in an entirely different order. His medical thinking was more like Mahoney's.

"Maybe this is a separate medical specialty."

Years later, Steinerman would recall this when he took the

accreditation exam, his changes in thought patterns essential to pass the rather rigorous written and oral certification exams.

Steinerman had to hand it to the thumbs up their asses for one thing, it was a good meeting overall.

Steinerman left on the last day of the meeting, but Mahoney stayed in New Orleans for an extra couple of days since Charity Hospital of Tulane University asked him to deliver several lectures to the new emergency medicine residents

Mahoney was in the men's room of the convention center when two well-known bloods came in to take a piss. They started talking, not realizing Mahoney was in one of the cubicles. They talked about residency-trained emergency physicians and what a problem they were becoming.

Mahoney could hear every word. Usually the "suits" spoke of such things in well-muffled stage whispers. A third crip came in, and related the story of a residency-trained "scrub" who'd opened a chest in one of his contract hospitals in L.A. The patient was an eighteen-year-old boy with a single stab wound to the chest which penetrated his heart.

"The 'scrub' opens his chest right there with a scalpel," the crip related, "and relieves the tamponade (a large blood collection around the heart literally strangling the heart, making death an imminent certainty unless the collection is decompressed), but the on-call surgeon goes bananas telling him, 'You opened it, you close it. You shouldn't be openin' chests in the emergency room anyhow. Only surgeons open chests.'

"Well, the residency-trained 'scrub' says, 'I didn't have twenty minutes to wait for you to drive in,' and they argue for awhile.

"Finally the surgeon comes in, and even though the kid survives the initial insult, he dies eight days later of resistant Pseudomonas. It's nobody's fault, the hospital's full of overprescribers, and the kid's immune system just ran out of steam. The surgeon who became the hero and gets his picture in the local newspaper for savin' the kid, now looks foolish.

"So he calls a meeting of the hospital's surgical committee, but the administrator tells them they can't officially state in writing the emergency physician can't open a chest because they're afraid if the Joint Commission or anybody else sees that in the hospital bylaws, the hospital might lose some reimbursement. However, the surgical committee wants it made clear if any emergency physician does it, they'll get replaced. So they solve their ridiculous 'turf problem' by taking the thoracotomy tray (an instrument tray necessary to open a chest) out of the emergency room, and mention to the O-J-T-er to get rid of the residency-trained doc cause they know he's going to take the fucking tray, and put it right back in the E.R.

"So then I get a call from the O-J-T-er who's been handed the problem by the surgical committee, and his solution is for ME to replace the director. I tell him that's going to be difficult, but the asshole reminds me my contract's up in June.

"I spent ten fucking thousand dollars moving this residency-trained 'scrub' from Cincinnati to L.A. because the O-J-T-er insists on a residency-trained director, and look what happens. Any of you guys got a residency-trained 'scrub' you can make a trade for?"

One of the bloods replied, "I'm also sick of these overqualified physicians. The residency-trained ones are too aggressive, too confident and smart-mouthed. They're more insistent that the cardiologists and orthopedists come in at night. They're even bothering the plastics' crowd. Right now I put that I want a residency-trained emergency physician in all my advertisements, and put a big ad in their job catalogue, but to tell you the truth, if I can get away with it, I don't hire them.

"As for the thoracotomy tray, just put the damn thing next to the fire extinguisher with a decal, 'In case of emergency, break glass.'"

Even Mahoney chuckled, giving himself away.

CHAPTER SEVENTEEN

MEA CULPA

"...mea maxima culpa."
—*The Confiteor*

Nuance means apprehension, but anxiety is an easy diagnosis. Anxiety borders on hysteria, exhibitionism, complaint, chronicity, and secondary gain. It's easily spotted by experienced nurses and clinicians.

Apprehension on the other hand is subtle, the fear, humiliation, jitteriness, unwillingness to leave the hospital one so desperately wants to leave. Apprehension means heart attack, bleeding tubal pregnancy, blood clot in the lung, ruptured aneurysm, that sense of impending doom the patient cannot articulate but only transmits, and it's only the best of physicians and largest of Cats that distinguish apprehension from anxiety. Medicare, Medicaid, Travelers, and the Blue Cross Prudent Buyer's Plans do not pay for the diagnosis of apprehension. HMO's don't believe in apprehension at all, or anxiety. Apprehension is a scent only the large Cats can smell, and when they do, there's usually blood, and unvesseled blood in a body cavity where it "ain't" supposed to be.

Steinerman saw Frederick Nightingale in the emergency department with substernal, oppressive chest pain, a pressure more than a pain. He'd just turned forty, didn't smoke, didn't drink, was thin, did have some high blood pressure, but certainly didn't fit the high-risk profile for a heart attack. Nightingale had just lost his uncle, who'd raised him as a child, and came to the emergency room with his closed fist on his chest, panting for air, begging for help, letting everyone know he was in a state of emotional distress.

Steinerman diagnosed him with hyperventilation, and sat down to talk to him. Nightingale's breathlessness disappeared, his heart rate dropped to normal, and his wife thanked Steinerman for his concern.

As Steinerman began to write discharge instructions, one of the nurses said, "Are you sure you want to do that?"

The large Cat instinctively changed his mind, ordering the whole nine yards: EKG, chest x-ray, cardiac enzymes, oxygen levels of the blood, and electrolyte values. They were all normal. He put Nightingale on a cardiac monitor for two hours, noting no irregularities. He gave him a sublingual nitroglycerin tablet, but nothing changed. The large Cat nurse had since gone home, and the patient was now anxious to leave himself, although he still had a twinge of pain. Steinerman discharged him, and the night nurse said as Nightingale left, "He looks apprehensive, Doctor Steinerman."

But the large Cat didn't click. No one knows why something mightn't click on a certain night. No night is ever a total washout. One never misses three things in a row, but on the best of nights in the best of months in the best of years, something, sometime, might not register even in the largest of Cats. It's not that one is inattentive, it's not that the sentry is lax on the watch that night, or has his or her mind on other things. One might catch the meningitis early or suspect the cooking appendicitis, one might pick up the glaucoma missed three days ago or scent the cyanosis. And for the obvious, one always get them. Thousands of correct diagnoses, thousands of proper treatments, hundreds of good choices in tough situations, scores of radio interventions to the paramedics, but on some nights in some areas for some reasons, things don't click, and doctors never hear the bullet hitting them.

They never hear it, only remember it for the rest of their lives, and the rest they forget. Nightingale's wife called back—her husband had stopped breathing.

Steinerman thought, "No, it couldn't be the five milligram Valium I gave him to help him sleep."

Steinerman followed the paramedic radio transmissions controlled by the General Hospital, the one closest to Nightingale's home, following the conversation until the paramedics arrived at the General, but Steinerman already knew the result.

Steinerman, the large Cat, always a troubleshooter, never minimizing a situation, a patient-centered, disciplined emergency physician who never let his guard down, simply didn't click that night.

Sheila Schultz was the Chief Medical Resident on duty at the General, directing Nightingale's resuscitation attempts. When it was over, she called Steinerman, opening with her charming brand of sarcasm, "I just wanted to give you some follow-up on the patient you saw and discharged three hours ago." The fucking little bitch went on to describe the cardiac arrest in detail and "all they did at the General, even though it too late." The senior medical resident hit Steinerman with her viciousness, ending the terse conversation with, "We just now pronounced him dead. Looks like you missed the big one."

One simple mishap and one creates a forty-year-old widow. One overreading creates a fatal allergic reaction in a nine year old, one underreading creates a motherless child. One little night when something doesn't click, and no one knows why, but it happens, and when it happens, there are very few physicians who openly extend the welcome to the club, the only club to which all physicians belong and don't want to.

Steinerman was devastated, and when he reviewed the case, it was such an obvious fuck up. Even the cardiogram, in retrospect, wasn't quite right. How could he have done that, he pondered. A malpractice suit didn't bother him; he was insured by Grand Bahamian, Inc. An invitation to Death and

Doughnuts? He could just sit there like Monk. But the consequences of one small mistake, one little error, the family devastations that occur when even the flawless game players like Abraham Steinerman don't click, and no one will ever know why.

Delorenzo called Steinerman, "I heard about the cardiac case. Remember, it's not been that long since you left the General to become a doctor in the real world without interns, residents, and fellows."

Delorenzo shared some of his experiences with Steinerman, his own homicidal experiences, both actively and passively, in the emergency department, telling him like Mahoney had, the experience would leave an empty hole inside him. He then gave Steinerman the best piece of medical advice to this day he'd ever received, "Don't take any time off, don't take any courses, don't read any journals, just get on the horse again, and make sure you work a good number of shifts in the next few weeks." The only remedy was to get on the horse and ride again.

Steinerman was officially welcomed to the club, and he never forgot Delorenzo for his kindness in calling. He'd met him only once, but obviously Mahoney had told Delorenzo about the mistake.

Those residency-trained Cats were something, a new breed on the horizon, but the poachers needed to be eliminated.

In fact, the poacher "suit" told Steinerman to take a three-day course in reading cardiograms, so that the "suit" could put the required piece of paper into his overstuffed file for the "quality assurance" program to legally protect the poacher, giving him a perfect paper trail for the future.

Asshole Walsh even called, telling Steinerman not to worry about it or be concerned, "It just happens."

Of course, if Steinerman were found with twenty-eight young boys buried in his basement, Fearless Frank Walsh would have still given him the same advice, "Things just happen, so don't worry about it." Walsh went on to give his own brand of advice.

"Find the cardiogram," Walsh suggested. "If it's abnormal, take it off the patient's chart and throw it away. It worked for me once. Without the abnormal cardiogram they'll have less of a case. I once blamed it on the EKG technician, and the hospital had to take the blame. It's better they fire a tech than your taking it on the chin there, Abe."

Steinerman thanked old "we never looked," cordially hanging up, but actually grateful to Walsh for calling him and trying, in his own way, Walsh's only way, to give Steinerman a boost. Steinerman, who thought he'd seen and heard it all, was stunned once again, but he was young and didn't realize doctors never stop stunning one another. Doctors enjoy stunning one other.

Steinerman was not in the best of mental condition when Dan Anderson called to tell him the news. In a lugubrious voice, Dan asked Steinerman to keep it quiet as Mahoney had obviously taken pains to keep the news secret. Dan had heard through the grapevine that Mahoney had accepted an offer from the General to begin an anesthesiology residency in the fall.

Mahoney was leaving emergency medicine to begin a career in anesthesiology, a not uncommon exit for young emergency practitioners who saw that the crips and the bloods had that stone wall up, making them pawns in the big "management" scheme for a good long time to come.

Every year a number of "scrubs" stopped pretending about their futures, doing another residency instead. The American Academy referred to these physicians as "burnouts." The sultan "suits," of course, never burned out, "managing" those contracts well into their Alzheimer years.

"It apparently came after the Hershey Medical Center announced it was disbanding the emergency medicine residency program," said Anderson.

Steinerman gasped, "What do you mean, Dan. They can't just disband a department. I mean you can't just say, o.k., let's have a medical school, but no more department of pediatrics. Or neurology. Are you sure about this, Dan?"

"Positive, Abe, it's officially dissolved. Phil took it pretty hard. Abe, you might as well face it, and think about moving on to something else while you're still young. Brokers' trafficking in physicians has now become institutionalized. You're going to have to pay a right-to-work fee to some 'suit' of whatever stripe forever, some 'suit' subleasing that one-twentieth of an acre on the hospital's first floor with a perpetual lien on your income, simply garnishing from your earnings. There're going to be no new kids on the block without a fight, and most likely, a federal law. You can't push that rock up the hill forever."

When Anderson hung up, Steinerman was as depressed as the time when Shelly died. He packed his bags to begin his trip to California, a working vacation.

CHAPTER EIGHTEEN

CALIFORNIA DREAMIN'

"Being unable to make what is just strong,
we have made what is strong just."
—*Pascal*

California. Fucking California. O my God, California. The crips and the fucking bloods of the east should come to California. Fucking California. Unbelievable California. It was so fucking unbelievable. The "suits" in California? O my God. Fucking California. Loch Ness monsters were the fucking minimum and O-J-T-ers were in short supply, having dropped like flies from all the vascular congestion of the Beluga and Perignon. Fucking California. The Visigoths and Vandals may have looted Rome, but it didn't compare with the sack by organized emergency medicine of the vast marketplace of California's emergency rooms. Getting a hundred grand or two for "managing" an emergency room in L.A. or a San Francisco suburb was the fucking minimum. It was incredible.

"Management" contracts of emergency departments in California were indeed a totally separate form of hard currency, like taxicab medallions, completely negotiable, highly marketable, eminently extortable, and always appreciating. Real estate values ran a poor second to an emergency medicine "management" contract in the providential promised land of California. No Black Mondays or distress sales in "management" in California because California was the fucking bull market of emergency medicine "management." Soda pop machines were everywhere, and there was a large blind spot for the highway robbery going on, the complete laissez-faire mentality, the trickle-down care for the populace, all on a munificent scale of economy in the unbelievable "management" mecca of California. Organized emergency medicine "management" had reached its apogee in California, and all the gold was there, making the weasels, crips, and bloods a fortuna bigger than a mountain of shit.

The "management" barrels of money also provided the "suits" with excellent housing, enormous haciendas at rather fine addresses with panoramic ocean and mountain views, because in their income bracket, it was as they sometimes say in California, affordable housing. No homeless "managers" in California. Oh, no, not in their income bracket, several homes were affordable. The "suits" in fucking California outbid the Japanese, the "suits'" income in California dwarfing the CEO's of banks, chip manufacturers, and commodity traders. Michael Milken and Ivan Boesky, step aside. The tax law did not apply to the California "suits," because they made so much money, they could simply pay their fucking taxes—local, state, federal, excise, FICA, property—and wipe out the fucking deficit with the change in their back pockets. Nothing in emergency medicine existed on quite the fucking scale it did in California. Forget AIDS, these poor patients in California needed a meningitis vaccine, and they needed one quick because petechiae might become a bigger crop than rice. Also, one might rhetorically add, California had the largest, most powerful and politically active state chapter of the American Academy of Emergency Physicians.

Steinerman began in Los Angeles, the City of Angels and a few Beelzebubs as well who'd found a very comfortable home in organized emergency medicine "management." Steinerman came to California because he'd originally signed a contract with Pyramid, Inc. to work in several states. Lyle had called for his pound of flesh, demanding Steinerman work a month in California. Steinerman didn't really mind, plus Eileen and Annie were coming out at the end of the third week.

There was one strange thing, however; Steinerman wasn't going to be working at a Pyramid, Inc. "managed" hospital since apparently Pyramid had lost the contracts at the hospitals where he was originally supposed to work. Pyramid, Inc., though, had subcontracted him to a fellow named Biggs.

Steinerman arrived a few days early, had some extra time in Los Angeles, and called Biggs. Since Biggs owned four "doc in the boxes" in the Los Angeles and Orange County areas, Steinerman thought he might need to fill in a blank or two. Biggs read Steinerman the credentials' riot act over the phone, telling him the standards were different for physicians who worked for him in fucking California.

"I only have the finest physicians work in my clinics. Are you board-accredited?"

"Yes, I'm certified in internal medicine."

"Not that, I mean emergency medicine."

"No, but I'm working on it. I have most of my hours accumulated."

"Well, yes, well, well, we certainly can't pay you as much money, but maybe we can use you part time, but only after you're proctored by one of my colleagues, of course. I should have known that fucking Lyle didn't have any board-accredited docs working for him. Well, where are you, I'll pick you up to discuss this."

It seemed rather strange Biggs was driving over to the hotel, but thirty minutes later Biggs arrived in his blue Porsche, and was on the car phone yelling, waving at Steinerman to get in.

Biggs saw that Steinerman was part of the white brotherhood—well dressed, didn't weigh four hundred pounds, and not sporting a pony tail—so he immediately planned to put him in his privately-owned Orange County Immediate Care Clinic, a "doc in the box." Biggs wasted no time hitting Steinerman like a locomotive, especially knowing Steinerman had come from Pyramid, Inc.

"You got your Advanced Cardiac and Trauma Life Support certifications?" He didn't give Steinerman a chance to answer. "Another thing, we don't care for graduates of foreign schools. This is California, young man, and we demand quality. We have the most rigorous credentialing policies of any state, and I know, because I wrote the policy for the California Academy of Emergency Physicians myself."

Suddenly the car phone rang, and Biggs turned bright red, screeching into the receiver, "This is the third goddamned time this month that jackass has called in sick! How the fuck can I staff these quack-in-the-shacks if you keep finding me these jokers. God damn it." He swung his fat reddened neck toward Steinerman. "Tonight? Can you work tonight?" Steinerman took the opportunity for a little amusement.

"I'd like to, but I guess I'd better tell you up front about my foreign medical school training."

"Forget that. Do you have a goddamned license?"

"Well, actually, its been reinstated."

"Is it an active, fucking unrevoked state medical license or not?"

"Oh yes, and I've agreed to..."

"I don't give a shit what you've agreed to do or not to do, and I don't give a shit what you did to lose your license in the first place. In fact, I don't want to know, so don't ever, ever tell me what it was. All I want to know, young man, is do you or don't you have an active legal license to practice medicine in the state of California? Yes or no! That's all I want to know!"

"Yes, but I've never been able to pass the Advanced Cardiac or Trauma Life Support courses, although I've taken them several times with my friend Doctor Monk."

"I know Monk, that fucking little homunculus. He's worked for me many times, and I specifically told Lyle not to send him as part of our deal either. You hang around with Monk? You don't look like his type! I don't know why he keeps going back to that fucking Pyramid, either. I've offered him more money than that cheap-ass, skinflint Lyle. Never mind that!" Biggs pulled over and took out a sheet of paper and started to write, "I... What the hell's your first name anyway?"

"Abe."

Biggs continued to write "I, Abe Stinman, M. D., possess an active, unrevoked medical license in the State of California."

"Sign this!"

As Steinerman was signing, Biggs whirled the Porsche around, immediately picking up the phone. He sped through two red lights screaming, "Don't worry about it. If we get stopped, we'll tell the highway patrol it's a medical emergency." They did stop at the third red light, and Biggs pulled out his briefcase, thrusting another paper at Steinerman to sign, the noncompete clause. "I almost forgot about this, it's important. Sign it and date it. We need this to maintain our quality. Also, sign this one too." The second one was a legally binding letter of confidentiality agreeing not to tell other physicians the hourly income Biggs was paying him.

Biggs had several physicians "on the run" working in his "doc in the boxes" so he paid them less. He didn't want other physicians telling the boys "on the run" how much they were making, not that it made much difference since the doctors "on the run" weren't inclined to return for another year in Saudi Arabia. Saudi is where the boys "on the run" worked for a year or two while their statute of limitations ran. Usually their justice problems were with federal authorities for transgressions involving income tax, child support, controlled drug overprescribing, and Medicare fraud, with an occasional murder.

Within twenty-five minutes, Steinerman was at work in the Immediate Care Clinic of Orange County.

Underneath the sign, "Immediate Care Clinic of Orange County," another sign read, "No Appointment Necessary," and underneath that, "***Quality*** Medical Care Provided by ***Quality*** Physicians." Mahoney was certainly right about the child abuse theory of non-owner occupied "doc in the boxes," and it was appallingly apparent to Steinerman that California was a big part of the epic joke. As Steinerman noted ***Quality*** pasted all over the windows of Biggs's "doc in the box," he knew, instead of the word ***Quality,*** what the clinic really needed was a warning stamp from the Surgeon General's office, or at least, "Parental Discretion Advised."

Steinerman called Mahoney, "Philip, I'm going to write a letter to the Academy telling them about California," but Mahoney warned his friend in the most serious of tones.

"Don't! I repeat, Abe, don't do it! California's a much bigger game, and those boys can give you a pretty loud leper bell! You've already been pinkslipped once for opening your mouth."

Mahoney went on to explain that California was nationally known as the home of the old-fashioned blackball in emergency medicine. "It was all started by a very famous weasel and prominent member of the Academy in Los Angeles County who'd gotten pissed off at several fine physicians who'd mutinied, demanding a fair share of the pie. The Los Angeles weasel created a blacklist that he shared with every major crip and blood in California. Abe, this Joe McCarthy-era enemies list can mean unemployment to the infidel in California. Many of the major groups cooperate, and several 'partnerships' mandate membership in the American Academy as a prerequisite for higher pay. Virtually all the major 'suits' in California stay on multiple committees, meeting regularly to 'work for the improvement of emergency-medical care,' but also to share dossiers and notes from the underground with one another on their private grapevine to form a closed shop if necessary. And don't forget, many of the letters to the Academy that end up in Kensington's landfill are anonymously postmarked from California cities. California emergency physicians were the first to realize, if you wrote a letter criticizing one of the major crips, bloods or weasels who were prominent members of the American Academy, it was a prudent thing not to sign your name."

Steinerman agreed to keep his mouth shut, going to work the next day in one of Bigg's "managed" emergency departments, just outside of Beverly Hills.

Steinerman was met with a very distant, cold reception from the nursing staff, both on the morning and evening shifts. The ice queens stayed frozen for the next few days, so one afternoon at lunch in the hospital cafeteria, Steinerman quizzed one of the black vocational nurses about the chill in the air.

"Well, it's quite simple," she quipped without batting an eye, "you're a scab."

"A scab?" the bewildered Steinerman asked. "What in the world do you mean I'm a scab? I'm just working a few shifts here for Biggs."

The pudgy, rolly-polly, night nurse who looked like a black Michelin Tire Man replied, "You're a scab, Doctor. You know very well that Doctor Biggs has to get rid of Doctor Anolik, our favorite doctor."

The unknowing Steinerman stared in disbelief. "Really," he said, "I really don't know what you're talking about. I'm not here to replace anybody. I had a contract to work for Pyramid which was subcontracted to Biggs, and that's why I'm here, and it's just for a few days. I don't even know this Anolik. Who is he and why is he leaving?"

"First of all, he's a she. Doctor Miriam Anolik is being forced out by Doctor Rubenstein, the orthopedist who hates her and all women. Secondly, it figures Doctor Biggs would do business with Pyramid. Our administrator threw Pyramid out of this hospital about a year ago. You never saw such creatures in your life as those things they call doctors comin' from that east coast Pyramid. I'd hate to get sick in Boston. They were just incredible. Why one of those doctors started hallucinatin' one night, and we had to call security to get him outta here. We still get letters in the mail from that crazy bird tellin' us it was our fault, and that we all planned it from the beginnin' to ruin his life. We told our head nurse we was all resignin', and goin' to the hospital cross town unless we stopped gettin' those east coast losers to work in our emergency room.

"One of our regular asthmatic patients was a writer for the Los Angeles Chronicle, and overhearin' us talkin' one day, he said he'd be happy to write a story about the whole thing for us, havin' a crush on Julie, one of our day nurses, at the time. That sure got 'em movin' and pretty soon they told us Pyramid was out."

Steinerman looked in the air for a minute feeling obliged to softly ask the rhetorical question, "Do you know Monk and Walsh?"

"O lordy, lordy, lordy, that Doctor Walsh. We had to go in and lift him right outta that bed, draggin' him in some nights to see patients. We hadda give him mouthwash and spray him down with perfumes and stuff to make him presentable smellin'. He was a mean one too, real mean, especially after drinkin' some of that foul smellin' stuff. They said it was real expensive scotch, but it smelled just like the dirt on my granddaddy's farm in North Carolina.

"What about Monk."

"He was a nice little guy never sayin' much, but like we used to say back home, he was dumber than a stump, 'Ozark Mountain Dumb,' as my cousins used to say. We used to haveta call to the pharmacy to change the medicines Doctor Monk prescribed to whatever the pharmacist thought best because Doctor Monk always used those new expensive medicines nobody's ever heard of. One of our heart surgeons from Atlanta told us to 'make sure we checked gizmo,' meanin' Doctor Monk 'to make sure he never had no Jarvik-7 in his briefcase,'" and she belly laughed, along with Steinerman.

"What about Doctor Anolik?" asked the chuckling Steinerman still thinking, "gizmo Monk with an artificial heart in his briefcase, now that's funny."

"Doctor Anolik is beautiful, just beautiful, but she don't take no lip from nobody and she sticks up for us, and that's what got her into so much trouble with Doctor Rubenstein, the bone doctor. He's always complainin' about everybody. But anyway, this Doctor Martin, our emergency room director, he writes everything down like a little old lady. They all had this meetin', and they said Doctor Anolik was to apologize to that old fool Doctor Rubenstein, and she says flat no, and so that's why they gettin' ready to fire her."

Steinerman knew the nurses were the most accurate source of information in any hospital's emergency room, especially the black vocational nurses with the twenty-year pins who worked the graveyard shift. They, like Mahoney, seemed to know everything, and were the group least in need of a lie detector test. So Anolik was fired because a misogynistic orthopedic surgeon, a Stullman from the Hopkins of sorts, complained about her, citing her "incompetence," and Martin crumbled.

Biggs knew what he had to do to maintain the "management" contract, and Biggs had to "maintain the contract." When Pyramid, Inc. was thrown out, Lyle informed Biggs that Anolik and Martin had two-year noncompete clauses. Since Pyramid had now been kicked out of virtually every California contract, they had no good will to lose in the state. Pyramid, Inc. made it clear they would vindictively create a legal nightmare for Biggs to "protect their interests," and Pyramid's "plea for injunction" might cause Biggs to lose his new "management" contract.

Biggs then agreed to pay twenty-five thousand dollars apiece for each of the noncompete clauses, another commodity in the business of emergency medicine, and he never mentioned the buyout to anyone. The buyout also required Pyramid, Inc. to find Biggs a generic physician for three weeks of transitional fill-in-the-blank coverage which Lyle was finally doing by sending Steinerman.

Anolik had to go, and the only way to get rid of her and appease the orthopod was to suggest, ever so subtly, that she look for a new job. Since Biggs had six "management" contracts in greater L.A., it was no problem, particularly since good "scrubs" were hard to find in L.A. He made her an offer she "couldn't refuse," the directorship of a nearby emergency room where the orthopod didn't have privileges, with a thirty-five thousand dollar a year directorship stipend, and no night shifts.

The thirty-five thousand dollar a year stipend to run one of the most difficult emergency rooms in Los Angeles County was a fair price, and should have been offered a long time ago to the previous director.

Also, Biggs left the innuendo to Anolik and her new fiance, who was sitting right there on the couch, that bone-crushing lawyers would pounce on Anolik if she refused to do it or if she pitched too big a stink.

That was a big mistake for Biggs because the thin, almost frail-looking young man sitting on the couch was Doctor Eric Manheimer, an internist with the largest population of well-insured elderly Jewish women this side of Tel Aviv.

Steinerman decided to go visit Anolik, meeting her for lunch on Rodeo Drive, an event known in L.A. as "doing lunch."

Anolik sat down, and Steinerman recognized those breasts as distinctive as Monroe's. He remembered Anolik from one disastrous night in an emergency room in Boston when a twenty-four year old woman, nine months pregnant arrived, essentially dead on arrival, after injuries sustained in an auto wreck. He and Mahoney were double covering, and they immediately performed a postmortem Caesarian-section, and paged over the hospital loudspeaker for any pediatrician to come to the emergency room STAT.

Under no legal obligation to respond, Doctor Anolik jumped into the pressure-cooker situation, and with her racehorse blood, she glovelessly took the baby, immediately placing a tube into her thick meconiom-stained trachea. The baby was clearly in fetal distress because prior to the C-section, the baby discharged its fetal fecal-contents called meconium, turning the normally crystal-clear amniotic fluid into a turbid, greenish-brown slurry with pebble-sized pieces of baby-shit, and the baby had aspirated some of the fluid into her airway.

Anolik screamed for suction and was handed the suction tube adapted to the tube she'd just placed, but the suction failed like it does many times in a crisis. Doctor Anolik then sucked out the meconium obstructing the airway with her own mouth, and after she sucked out a full mouthful of babyshit, the child began to breath.

The neonate spent a month in the ICU, eventually graduating from the nursery with a normal I.Q.

Steinerman joyously said, "I remember you! You're the one who sucked the meconium out of the baby's mouth during the disaster. What are you doing in Los Angeles?"

Anolik laughed, having remembered the handsome Steinerman herself, and said, "You know the saying, 'Go West, young woman.'" Steinerman laughed, and bluntly stated his desire to learn why she was being fired.

Anolik took out a piece of paper with a list of the pros and cons of her leaving because of the orthopedic woman hater, the list drawn up for her by the well-meaning Martin. Steinerman thought how strange for a director to make up a list of the "pro" and "con" aspects of her being fired.

On the "con" side it mentioned the "stability of the contract" was being jeopardized, and that it would "set a bad precedent" (also on the con side) if it was too visible why she was leaving. This would encourage other staff physicians to try to do away with their least favorite emergency physician by bitching to Martin and Biggs, and doctors love to bitch.

The paper also suggested she try to "do lunch" with the orthopod, offering the olive branch, and getting more involved with any doctor with whom she might not be "communicating" effectively.

Miriam Anolik was a superlative clinician and a generously spirited woman, but like Delorenzo, she was clearly not an "effective communicator," but instead a bluntly honest woman, something the patients of Beverly Hills desperately needed.

Elderly women develop a fairly characteristic set of age-related diseases, namely cataracts, osteoporosis, arthritis, and gastrointestinal bleeding from the arthritis medicines.

The orthopedic surgeon makes twenty-five hundred dollars to repair a broken hip, thirty-five hundred if he or she has to replace the entire hip joint, the ophthalmologist fifteen hundred to replace an opacified, cataratic lens with a clear implant, and the gastroenterologist six-hundred dollars to flashlight a bleeding patient.

Although the general internist netting a hundred grand a year actually works the hardest, he or she is at the bottom of the totem pole when it comes to reimbursement, and the internists and the family practitioners usually work themselves into a massive coronary with a quadruple bypass by the age of fifty-five. Radiologists, by the way, tend to die at an old age of "natural causes."

The internists' and family practitioners' only justice is that the subspecialists all rely heavily upon them for referrals. A busy primary-care doctor with a well-insured patient population can make a significant boost to a procedural subspecialist's tax bracket.

Eric Manheimer was a superlative internist, *the* internist in the Brentwood area, a compulsive worker with a large, stable, geriatric practice of well-heeled patients inherited from his retired father's medical practice, and he had not accepted new patients in over a year. Each year, four per cent of his osteoporotic patients fell, breaking their hips, and he referred them to the orthopedic group of Rubenstein, Sobol, Lite and Lite.

Manheimer's younger brother, Joshua, was a pediatrician in the area, having a large practice of actively overachieving teenagers who regularly broke their elbows, ankles, and occasionally their femurs during football skirmishes. He also referred to the Rubenstein group.

When the Manheimer-Anolik engagement was announced, another announcement of sorts was posted in the emergency department.

From: Eric Manheimer, M.D., Diplomat American Board of Internal Medicine
Joshua Manheimer, M.D., Diplomat American Board of Pediatrics

To: Emergency Department, Cedar Mountain Hospital

Re: All orthopedic cases from our practice will no longer be referred to Doctors Rubenstein, Sobol, Lite and Lite. Regarding all orthopedic referrals, we wish to be paged. If one of our patients specifically requests the above group, please call us at our unlisted numbers. Doctor Eric 344-5623, Doctor Joshua 344-6739.

To say the shit hit the fan from this unusual posting of the Manheimers would be an indescribable understatement. The shock wave emanating from the epicenter of the Cedar Mountain Hospital shook the Brentwood-Beverly Hills medical community so hard it almost fell into the Santa Monica Bay.

Manheimer's office was deluged with calls from procedural subspecialists hoping they had done nothing to offend the brothers Manheimer or the brothers Manheimer's partners, excellent physicians themselves with a large well-insured patient referral base.

Usually the rheumatologist, Corey Partridge, didn't complain about such things, since Pyramid, Inc. knew by the time an excellent internist referred him a patient, he or she'd already blown the therapeutic wad, leaving Partridge with no easy tricks up his sleeve. However, there was a great deal of concern amongst the doctors, even Partridge, on this matter because everyone had always found Anolik a fine clinician who was very cordial to their patients, and regularly had her on their social invitation and holiday gift list.

They also knew Rubenstein could be an asshole, but it seemed incomprehensible that Rubenstein, or any other physician, could get another physician thrown out. They concluded that with someone as fine as Anolik, it was impossible, totally impossible.

They felt this way, of course, because they were unfamiliar, as were virtually all practicing physicians in all specialties other than emergency medicine, with the "contract" and "management" groups and the "noncompete clauses."

They were mildly aware that the philosophy of the American Academy of Emergency Physicians had a strong wink-and-nod attitude toward some unsavory practices, but this was something out of Kafka. They, like Dan Anderson's staff doctors, weren't about to believe anything like this could possibly exist in American medicine.

They concluded something else must be cooking, maybe the Manheimers had become Jews for Jesus or something horribly bizarre had happened to them. After all, they did both work very hard for relatively little money. Maybe they'd just snapped? They were both pissed off at something or somebody, but what and why?

But the staff doctors would never know the real answer, and were somewhat validated in their original thinking because, as it turned out, Doctor Miriam Anolik wasn't fired after all.

It was certainly an amusing sight for all to witness Rubenstein coming down to the emergency room every afternoon with his hospital cafeteria tray for two to "do lunch" with Doctor Anolik.

O, how the mighty can fall sometimes. Rumor had it that Elaine Sobol, and Scott and Shelly Lite were actively disengaging from Rubenstein, Sobol, Lite and Lite and, in fact, all clinicians receiving referrals from the Manheimers were distancing themselves quite visibly in the doctors' lounge from their old buddy Rubenstein.

Rumor also had it, if Anolik were fired, she might join the Manheimers in their medical practices, and start accepting new patients, generating even more subspeciality referrals which scared the shit out of everyone even more.

But Miriam was not without her pride. She told the inundated administrator she would stay only if they made her the director of the emergency department, which Rubenstein enthusiastically supported. Since Rubenstein was on the executive committee of the hospital, he personally called the shocked Biggs to tell him his "management" contract would not be renewed if Doctor Anolik wasn't made the director of the emergency room.

Biggs protested, "But last week you told me you weren't going to renew my contract unless I got rid of her. Now you're saying you won't renew my contract unless I keep her, and make her the director? What the hell's going on here?"

Rubenstein forcefully said, "Last week I was mistaken, and now she stays and is made the director, or we'll give the contract to someone who will do it."

Biggs was furious, but knew he couldn't piss Rubenstein off, so he immediately agreed to do it. Not only did Biggs have to give Anolik that thirty-five thousand dollars a year raise to be the director, but he also had to "bribe" Martin with another thirty-five grand to be the director of his other hospital.

It took Biggs two months to make up the loss of fifty grand for the commodities and then seventy on top of that, so he paid the newly-graduated emergency physicians less money to work weekend night shifts to offset the buyouts, keeping his own income unchanged. Biggs learned, like Goldman and Lyle, that emergency medicine in nineteen-ninety-two was a fucking bitch, and that he was worth every penny of his "management" money.

CHAPTER NINETEEN

THE EMPIRE STRIKES BACK

"I've got a family to support, and I can't
afford to tell the whole truth."
—*Mark Twain*

When things worked in medicine, it's amazing how well they did work, and trauma centers, like burn units and poison-control centers, worked.

Although it's uncertain the full constellation of factors enabling their incredibly successful operation, the central concept was dedicated centers where nurses and doctors saw only trauma patients brought in directly from the scene of an accident.

It grew out of the rapid transportation era of Vietnam when surgeons brought home the concept of the "Golden Hour," saving many an American life. It was in the "Golden Hour" that patients needed to be resuscitated or they lapsed into irreversibility, and like most advances in surgery, it evolved out of warfare.

In World War I, surgeons took home the experience of amputation, in World War II, blood transfusions, and in the Korean Conflict, rapid transport.

The Vietnam-era surgeons brought home the concepts of paramedic field stabilization, airway placement, and restoration of effective, circulating blood volume while en route to a center that sees only trauma victims, and where the trauma team doctors, surgical nurses, and ancillary staff are already in place, waiting for the patient. The patient never waits for the doctors, the doctors wait for the patient. The Vietnam-era surgeons took everyone a long way from the white to black Cadillacs.

The "suits" initially descended upon trauma centers with their true predatory instincts, while hospital administrators made bids so their hospital, and not the one next door, would become the designated, regional trauma center winning all the prestige that went with it. It was felt the hospital would generate more business by this community-wide designation as paramedics were instructed to bypass hospital facilities closer to the accident scene, transporting patients to a designated trauma center, even if it was several miles out of their way. Every O-J-T-er was on the bandwagon in the late seventies and early eighties.

Norman Lyle was in the great City of London in the early eighties studying regionalized trauma centers, looking for another arena of emergency medicine to parasitize, but he had the same recurring thoughts, remembering those early lean years when he was still one of the "scrubs."

Lyle simply disliked victims of trauma, and in fact, felt he'd met a better class of people hitchhiking. Everyone in Boston that had gotten shot or stabbed pretty much deserved it, along with the car-accident crunchies always caused by drunks, and those freedom-loving idiots on their "murdercycles" and "Hondacides" without helmets.

He realized another reason why he disliked trauma victims so much—virtually none of them had any medical insurance. Lyle was never crazy about indigent souls of any kind, nothing making him more bilious than an injured welfare mother giving birth to an uninsured baby.

Then it hit Lyle, "These trauma centers are going to suffer huge monetary loses. They aren't enlarging their facilities, and trauma patients are going to use up all the resources, blood, and operating-room time. They're going to tie up intensive-care-unit beds, taking the beds away from paying heart attacks and medically-ill patients. The head-injured will tie up the neuro units for weeks," and indeed, it was a farsighted Lyle who steered clear of hospitals with active Level One trauma centers, aiming his glossies at the surrounding Level Two hospitals.

His predictions, which he kept to himself, were borne out, and starting in Los Angeles, hospitals in the late nineteen eighties stampeded in a mad rush to get themselves downgraded from Level One Trauma Centers to Level Two Centers. Level Two centers did not require a group of dedicated traumatologists, only an orthopedist and a general surgeon who agreed to stay sober for twenty-four hours of call.

Also, although not common, the general surgeon on call in the Level Two centers occasionally stalled through the entire "Golden Hour" before answering his emergency-room page.

The Level Two hospitals and their administrators were quite happy to wave at the Econolines passing their institutions on the way to the more prestigious and poorer hospitals. So in a way, with the crips, bloods, and weasels redlining the unprofitable trauma centers, along with burn units and poison-control centers, the seriously traumatized, burned, and poisoned patients received much better care.

Steinerman hadn't worked in any of the Level One, regionalized trauma centers in California since Biggs also avoided them.

The following week, Eileen and Annie arrived. They spent some time with Eileen's ex-in-laws, and scouted the Southern California region one more time for a possible place to settle, but all knew they were quite content in Boston.

Although it was hard to believe any group of people could be a less responsible lot than the citizenry of Boston, Steinerman realized the great unwashed of California really did push the envelope. Californians had the attitude, "Grandma's constipated again. Joey, dial 911. Why fight the traffic?" Econolines clogged the toll-free lanes of the highways in California stretching the overburdened and underfunded 911 system. And so, Steinerman, Eileen, and Annie took to the friendly skies returning to Boston, quite happy to be home. The next day he called Mahoney.

"Philip, when I was leaving California, I heard there were at least two dozen 'suits' making over three quarters of a million dollars every year without seeing any patients themselves. It seems to me there are several 'suits' with their hands in this extra-sweet cookie jar in gross violation of the Seventh Commandment of God. How do they manage to openly operate within the law?"

"It's pretty simple, Abe, there are no laws. Speaking of the Seventh Commandment, Abe, I'm having a problem with Goldman. I'm not sure what's going to happen, but I'll keep you posted. Good to have you guys back in town. I'll see you next week, and we'll see you all at Thanksgiving dinner."

Mahoney had worked at Braintree Children's Hospital for a little over two years, and was now the director, still working for Goldman's group. He and Tahoe had their home there, their daughter enrolled in a progressive local pre-school, and Tahoe was pregnant with their second child. The hospital was a well-known pediatric institution and a regional, cystic-fibrosis center.

Goldman's contract hinged upon Mahoney's overall competence and ability to create sociability, but Mahoney's single anchor wasn't enough. Goldman's Goldmanites proved too much for the administrator and the local pediatricians, many of them subspecialists, many of them foreign medical graduates with much higher standards than the Goldmanites.

The administrator told Brother Goldman his contract would not be renewed.

The new group replacing Goldman's "management" was an excellent, six-member physician group, all residency trained, and two were from Boston Children's Hospital. The board of directors of Braintree Children's, a rather erudite group of volunteers, was proud this newly-formed emergency medicine group chose Braintree in which to live and work. The administrator was well aware he wouldn't have to bother with the crips, bloods, pledge drivers, mosquitoes, sidekicks, Pinnacleites or Goldmanites again, just competent physicians forming an honestly-managed emergency team. The O-J-T-er also made it clear he didn't want any more Beluga, Loch Ness Monsters, Chardonnay, Perignon, or Red Sox tickets, nor did he want the emergency physicians in local shopping malls on weekends taking blood pressures in front of Sears department stores, nor did he want any of the other fruitcake "products" and "services" Pyramid, Inc. and Hospital Concessionaires of America, Inc. kept pushing. So the promotional Brother Goldman was given the bum's rush out of Braintree Children's, but the new group and the hospital administrator wanted the experienced and well-respected Mahoney to remain the director.

Goldman was furious with this humiliating loss right on his front doorstep, the hospital being less than three miles from his home and main office, a stinging embarrassment. He immediately started notifying local physicians and hospitals, saying, "I'm relieved not to service this difficult hospital any longer. I've been losing over twenty thousand dollars a year on that sinkhole," but he desperately wanted to get even with those parvenus, especially the residency-trained ones. He put the mosquitoes, pledge drivers, sidekicks, red pins, start-up-set-up physicians, and other members of his emergency medicine dignity battalions on it.

As it turned out, Mahoney had worked there for the past two years, was then made the director, continuing to work at Children's under a standard contract as the director of the emergency department, except that Tahoe had crossed out the two-year noncompete clause, writing in six months.

Goldman went through his files enraged that the two-year

noncompete had been lined through restraining Mahoney from working at Children's for only six months. Goldman stewed in almost uncontrollable anger, especially because of rumors from the Academy that Kensington was writing an encyclical defending the various mini-empires organized emergency medicine was creating. All the "suits" would be talking about how he'd been dethroned at Children's, and in the postmortem, many crips and bloods would have a field day changing the yellow pins on Goldman's hospitals to red ones.

Goldman remembered the pledge drivers were desperate at the time to fill in some blanks, and now he could sandbag Mahoney coming and going for only six months. After Mahoney stayed away from Braintree Children's for six months, he'd be a free agent, and could return as the director. Goldman knew his empire had to mercilessly strike back at Mahoney.

He called Mahoney, warning him of the arsenal of legal artillery at his disposal, and that he would pursue every legal weapon to preserve his contract rights, pulverizing Mahoney with a bankrupting litigation nightmare.

But Mahoney reminded Goldman of his interest in cystic fibrosis, asking to be released from the noncompete clause since it was only for six months. He explained how he knew the backgrounds of many of these children, especially the very-ill ones who frequented the emergency department. He also pointed out winter was approaching, causing an abrupt increase in emergency admissions in the kids with cystic fibrosis, and he could be an invaluable service to the new group.

Goldman scoffed with contempt at Mahoney's flagrant disregard of the marketplace and the sanctity of the contract. His voice was full of hair-raising bellicosity, demonstrating his fury at Mahoney for even the merest consideration of not adhering to the most sacred principle of the theocracy called the American Academy of Emergency Physicians, its central canon, its raison d'etre, the contracts of the "suits" with their sacrosanct noncompete clauses.

The blasphemous Mahoney got the same Dick and Jane

history lesson of free enterprise that Adkins got on how Goldman had "risked his own money," Goldman not thinking for a minute about his tremendous dividend on Mahoney already, even for the bluest of chips.

Goldman simmered down, recovering his gentler, conciliatory business tone, telling Mahoney he had to do this so as "not to set an unhealthy precedent in the climate of emergency medicine."

Mahoney knew he didn't have the resources or support to fight Goldman.

Goldman was being evicted from the "management" contract at Children's Hospital because he'd hired too many understudies for real emergency physicians, but his top-flight legal department took a back seat to no one, and Mahoney knew Goldman would kneecap him with that litigation nightmare in a heartbeat. Goldman warned Mahoney that contract law afforded Hospital Concessionaires of America, Inc. ironclad protection with little room for "scrub" maneuvering in spite of the public good.

Goldman was practical, though, telling Mahoney a race to the courthouse would be suicide for Mahoney as well as a needless expense for himself. He offered Mahoney another hospital an hour away that had some staffing problems, since his main start-up physician had just defected to one of Pyramid, Inc.'s new flagships for more money. Mahoney hesitated, but Goldman offered commuting expenses as well, so he just shrugged. What could he do?

"I'll be out of emergency medicine," the resigned Mahoney told Steinerman that night, "and into anesthesia soon enough. Besides, I have a family to support now, so I've got to cotton to Goldman for a couple of months."

The next day he capitulated, signing with Goldman's emergency medicine "management" team for the new hospital. Goldman was personally there, making sure the apostate Mahoney and his smart-alec wife didn't line out the two-year noncompete clause of the over-punctuated contract.

Unbeknownst to Mahoney at the time, Goldman had called the administrator at Braintree Children's to ask if he really wanted Mahoney to stay on as the director. The administrator was quite pleased saying, "Of course. We and the new group of pediatricians and emergency physicians would love to have Doctor Mahoney stay on as our director, and Doctor Goldman, that's quite generous of you to offer, and I shall not forget it."

But the heavy-cheeked Goldman wasn't a generous man, and had a murkier motive in mind saying, "Fine, but it will cost you fifty thousand dollars to buy out Doctor Mahoney's noncompete clause."

The stunned administrator gasped saying, "No, thank you," and hung up because the O-J-T-er couldn't stomach him any longer, and never wanted anything to do with scuzzball Goldman or his brown-shirted mosquitoes again.

CHAPTER TWENTY-ONE

THE ONE HUNDRED AND EIGHTY THOUSAND DOLLAR PAIR OF SUNGLASSES

"Some physicians feel that they should be able to charge the patients that way. And that is something which is contrary to the free enterprise, competitive, economic system under which we live. For example, a pair of eyeglasses is worth tens of thousands of dollars to me. But the cost of that pair of eyeglasses is maybe $80. We do not let the eyeglass makers charge us $20,000 for a pair of eyeglasses. Because that would be unfair practice. In medicine, that may not work very well, because when you and I become seriously ill, if our life is threatened we're not going to shop around. So, in that sense, you see, medicine holds some monopolistic power."

—William Hsiao, Ph.D., Professor of Economics and Health Policy, Harvard School of Public Health Director, Resource-Based Relative Value Scale Study

Reviewing the Goldman Enterprises,

Trauma Specialists, Incorporated
Acute Care Specialists, Incorporated
Pediatric and Trauma Systems, Incorporated
Pediatric and Toxicology Specialists, Incorporated

Emergency Care Medical Group, Incorporated
Emergency Medical Care Group, Incorporated
Emergency Group Medical Care, Incorporated
Emergency Physicians, Incorporated
Emergency Medical and Surgical Care Specialists, Incorporated
Emergency Surgical and Medical Care Specialists, Incorporated

Of New England, a wholly owned subsidiary of:

Pediatric Emergency Care, Incorporated
Trauma Specialists, Incorporated
Acute Care Specialists, Incorporated
Pediatric and Trauma Systems, Incorporated
Pediatric and Toxicology Specialists, Incorporated
Emergency Care Medical Group, Incorporated
Emergency Medical Care Group, Incorporated
Emergency Group Medical Care, Incorporated
Emergency Physicians, Incorporated
Emergency Medical and Surgical Care Specialists, Incorporated
Emergency Surgical and Medical Care Specialists, Incorporated

Of The Empire State, a wholly owned subsidiary of:

Pediatric Emergency Care, Incorporated
Trauma Specialists, Incorporated
Acute Care Specialists, Incorporated
Pediatric and Trauma Systems, Incorporated
Pediatric and Toxicology Specialists, Incorporated
Emergency Care Medical Group, Incorporated
Emergency Medical Care Group, Incorporated
Emergency Group Medical Care, Incorporated
Emergency Physicians, Incorporated
Emergency Medical and Surgical Care Specialists, Incorporated
Emergency Surgical and Medical Care Specialists, Incorporated

Of the Middle Atlantic States, a wholly owned subsidiary of:

Pediatric Emergency Care, Incorporated
Trauma Specialists, Incorporated
Acute Care Specialists, Incorporated
Pediatric and Trauma Systems, Incorporated
Pediatric and Toxicology Specialists, Incorporated
Emergency Care Medical Group, Incorporated
Emergency Medical Care Group, Incorporated
Emergency Group Medical Care, Incorporated
Emergency Physicians, Incorporated
Emergency Medical and Surgical Care Specialists, Incorporated
Emergency Surgical and Medical Care Specialists, Incorporated

A wholly owned subsidiary of

Hospital Concessionaires of America, Incorporated

with one voting shareholder

David Goldman, M. D.

Now that the infrastructure of the Emergency Medicine Industrial Complex was operating throughout the United States of America, many wondered about the academics.

"Do they also have their heads up their asses?" asked Steinerman one day.

Mahoney replied, "It's more like they keep their heads in the ozone. They seem to take pride in the fact they don't know what's going on, but as far as I can tell, none of them are actively involved in the scams. On the other hand, they've never had any outcry so I guess they really do love their blindfolds."

"But why," Steinerman asked, "doesn't somebody tell the emergency residents what awaits them outside of academia? Why have them apprentice for four years, filling their heads full of false expectations, only to inform them that the keys to the kingdom have been stolen? Why not at least give them a signpost or two before letting them get shanghaied? What's wrong with the academics, anyhow?

"Abe, you know it's impossible for five or six graduating residents with a totally desynchronized sleep pattern to travel all over creation to find a suitable emergency room to staff. There are no war rooms in the residency programs. Besides, the residents can't afford the Beluga or the Superbowl seats," both taking a minute to laugh.

"The con men spend their entire working day pursuing contracts, having whole staffs under them biting administrators daily. How the hell can we generate a power base like theirs while we're shell shocked nightly in the middle of the residency program? You know how difficult it is to keep your bearings after staying up several nights in a row, let alone market yourself against major corporations."

"Phil, you're still not answering my question," Steinerman said with a note of irritation. "I want to know why the academics tolerate these fraudulent washouts of rotating internships who now openly describe themselves as the Daniel Boones of emergency medicine, aligning themselves with the faculties, and the dumbshit faculties aligning themselves right along with the 'suits.' It seems to me it was the academics who legitimized emergency medicine, making it into an accepted specialty, but now they deliver the residents bound hand and foot over to a group of pizza executives and soda machine owners. Why do the academics suddenly act like the head injured when the subject of these kitchen scheduling clowns comes up? You know, Anderson is right. This specialty is the laughingstock of hospital administrators. Everyone knows large corporations on the New York Big Board are trying to buy shares in the lucrative emergency medicine 'management' marketplace. Are the academics going to let the promising specialty die of internal injuries? What the hell is the matter with them, Phil?"

Mahoney replied, "The academics and the thumbs up their

asses have actually achieved a miracle of sorts, Abe. Through their acrobatic avoidance of difficult ethical issues, they've managed to stick their whole heads up their asses. It would take Cro-Magnon with his scope to find their heads, and even if he found them, it would take forceps with the clench of a pit bull to pull their reluctant heads out to see the world as it really is." Mahoney told Steinerman to give it up, "Don't rock the boat any more. They're a big outfit, Abe, backed by some pretty rich people, rich people with a lot to lose."

Steinerman wondered, rather surprised the omniscient Philip Mahoney had no better explanation than that.

Many answers lay in the alchemy of transforming the clinical dollars of hands-on doctors into "management" money, the handsome, twenty-five per cent or more of the gross Norman Lyle hatched in that epochal picosecond on the sugar frosted flakes counter.

In so-so neighborhoods with poor patient-payer mixes, the numbers boiled down to about fifty dollars an hour, round the clock, throughout the year. Some of the slumlord weasels, crips and bloods made a little less than that, but the general rule of thumb was the "rule of fifteens." A "suit" would take home fifteen thousand dollars a month as Caesar's due for "managing" an emergency room seeing about fifteen thousand patients a year, and it takes him less than fifteen hours a month to kitchen schedule, and keep the whole "quality assurance" and "risk management" thing going. Once this little principality is set on autopilot, relatively easy to do in any large city, it becomes the eighth financial wonder of the world.

That was the lure attracting so many misfits and born deceivers, and not a few unbalanced individuals, to be the contract holders with the hospitals to "manage" the emergency rooms in a true, top-down, totalitarian sheikdom.

Fifteen thousand smackers a month is actually on the low side, existing in relatively poor areas. With wealthier patient-payer mixes, the cherrypicking "suits" could easily make seventy to a hundred dollars an hour round the clock, receiving more than four-hundred-thousand big ones a year for "managing" one emergency room.

But when those physicians making huge sums of money off of the sweat of other physicians sat in the doctors' morning coffee lounge, they faced anesthesiologists, internists, pediatricians, radiologists, gynecologists, child psychiatrists, surgeons, neurosurgeons, vascular surgeons and orthopedists. Every one of these physicians makes money the old fashion way, by seeing sick and injured patients. In that doctors' coffee lounge there is one, and only one fat cat, making over a quarter of a mill a year clear profit by kitchen scheduling in one the cleverest scams ever developed.

Since no physician can justify the fifteen thousand dollars a month for fifteen hours scheduling time, now called "management," they can't look at other physicians directly in the eye, so the "suits" have to look at other physicians through sunglasses, their fifteen thousand dollars a month, or their annual one-hundred-and-eighty-thousand-dollar pair of sunglasses.

The only problem the "suits" had was looking over their shoulders for the Pyramids and Goldmans who so desperately wanted that quarter mill for themselves, to fend off the so-called "contract runs" every year when renewal time comes up. Who would have ever believed this one small step for the "suits," and one giant leap backward for mankind could have ever occurred in American medicine? No wonder they fired Dan Anderson.

Steinerman had by now met many crips, bloods, and weasels. He noted funny things happened to the men themselves of sudden, lottery-winner wealth, gouged from the fees of physicians actually treating the patients. These fast-buck artists first developed a peculiar xenophobia, best described as a stockpiling mentality, stuffing their mattresses with dollars. But after they hoarded enough rainy-day funds, they, like Lyle, began to develop the ache, finding it necessary to become men of good taste as well. Many succumbed to *The Last Temp-*

tation, terribly desirous of what rich men in the last third of their lives covet the most—respectability and dignity. The gloating "suits" found it distasteful to discuss something so vulgar as money, preferring the word fairness, bloody fairness, as these men of sudden culture, now acculturated to easy dollars, forgot they were a group of common vandals.

Even more peculiar things happened to the craftier men of emergency medicine commerce making twenty-five thousand dollars a month take home pay in the big "management" scheme. These gentlemen farmers of emergency medicine hyperventilated at the thought of doing another rectal exam, and unlike trauma surgeons, didn't want to expose themselves to HIV-positive blood, especially when they were dressed in evening clothes attending banquets honoring each other. They became stranger and stranger, beginning to reread the words of Francis Peabody, William Osler, and the Sermon on the Mount.

Uncle Max wasn't given to humanistic phrases, and the "suits" didn't care to read about bone marrows, so Uncle Max wasn't part of the required reading after one was fattened up on the storage disease of twenty-five thousand dollars a month of after expenses "management" money.

The gentrified "suits" began to understand "the secret of caring for the patient" on a more subtle plane than the "scrubs," giving moving lectures at national meetings on what it meant to doctors like Miriam Anolik. As the born-again "suits" studied the old goats Osler and Peabody, they also stimulated their beta-endorphins with new editions of contract-law books, and began to enjoy the profits from their soda machines on a subtler level as well, but felt more and more like fish out of water in the emergency room itself, and more and more persnickety about those rectal exams.

Instead, they preferred to participate visibly in a wide variety of civic, religious, and humanitarian projects with members of the *Social Register* trying to bury that old skinhead image.

Men, sucking twenty-five grand a month off the top from the fees of the conscripts, also began to write. They wrote letters of outrage to the Journal of Rabbit Brain Death concerning seatbelts, gun control, and airbags, desiring to write chapters of scholarly merit in textbooks as well. They told practicing physicians to be more tolerant of and look more beatifically at the (insured) huddled masses, and in addition, to take care of themselves, not to buy a home that's too expensive, to exercise, and develop therapeutic hobbies. They liked to sit back in that easy chair like Lyle in London saying fuddy-duddy, sappy, humanistic things to the world.

Many of the original Saville Row "suits" were now fifty-something, very rich but somewhat crotchety, and in spite of their personal trainers, a little flabby, with the more risky abdominal obesity pattern. They became very conscious of their middle age, their diet-controlled diabetes, and their name in print. The memoirists fretted over their standing in the pantheon of leaders in the storybooklike history of emergency medicine which they were now (re)writing like taxidermists, removing all the blots. Instead of honorably dying in obscurity with a burial at sea, some of the self-mythologizing goodfellas were videotaping themselves, looking like a group of stuffed animals for posterity.

The men who were making in excess of twenty-five thousand dollars a month, many very active in the running of the Academy, began to act even more funny. The formerly wealth-driven "suits" no longer had to fight the rear guard actions against the other crips and bloods. Many were in cahoots now, and because of their Pax Romana, didn't send glossies to each others' hospitals. They began to feel *The Call of the Wild* that many before them had felt. Like Lyle, they had that "willingness to serve" mentality crop up again, and it was that itch-to-serve mentality that was becoming the most dangerous aspect of the delivery of emergency care in America.

The "suits" coalesced, recycling their love-of-the-eighties money into Pyramidology fellowships in a bizarre partnership with the heads in the ozone academics, who themselves were now feeding antidepressants to the rabbits before Vaselining them and whacking them to death, and publishing the data in the Journal of Rabbit Brain Death.

More importantly, some of the very rich "suits" went completely off their rockers, running for public office. This represented the most pernicious threat to the state of emergency-medical care, "suits" in public office at any level.

It behooved the "suits" to keep a tenured "scrub" at the same hospital to placate the O-J-T-ers who were getting more sophisticated in reading wine lists. However, in reality, lifer "scrubs" usually began to cause trouble after four or five years. If they weren't trapped by houses, two bad marriages, or several whole-life insurance policies, they would move on after a short scuffle with the Goliaths looking for a more equitable share of the pie.

However, many were trapped, and resignation was the most adaptive response. But the "scrubs" knew the honest graft of the crips and the bloods was way out of line for the minimalist and many times destructive "products" and "services" the "suits" provided.

The "scrubs" also knew, besides fattening up the con men, every hour they worked, a portion of their fees went to fund the war chest to bankroll more glossies, more pledge drivers, more mosquitoes, more and increasingly tricky "quality assurance" forms to be filled out for form's sake, more green pins, more Beluga, and more playoff-payoff tickets while they funded the whole perversion of the newly formed, but deformed commodity called organized emergency medicine, still drifting kitchenwards.

It was certainly odd what a quarter of a mill for a job requiring only thirty thou could do to a group of non-physician M.D.s over a period of ten to twenty years. It seemed to be at that five million dollar mark of net wealth when the strange behavior began. At the twenty million dollar high-water mark of net kitchen scheduling wealth, a strange contagious vocabulary developed, and sometimes the "suits" had to sit near each other so they could communicate because the languages began to diverge. By not seeing patients, the "suits" had developed a communal form of cabin fever. Their money lingo was spoken in the hyperarticulate, pentecostal tongues of Laffer Curves, Managerial Grid, Theory Z, G-7, *The One Minute Manager,* pork bellies, a return to the gold standard, and the deficit, oh, the deficit. Nothing seem to rankle the "suits" more than the federal deficit.

In fact, the Academy's meetings had to be separated into a clinical track and a separate "management" track, held in separate rooms, the original dichotomy of "suits" and "scrubs" becoming a visible chasm with the big "management" meetings held at the most expensive hotels and resorts.

Mahoney once mentioned to Goldman he was thinking of going to the annual "management" meeting.

Goldman turned in disbelief as if Mahoney had gone off the deep end, and said, "You know the rooms are a hundred and seventy dollars a night?"

CHAPTER TWENTY-TWO

UNCLE HERSHEL'S VISIT

"God is on the side of the largest army."
—*Napoleon*

Mahoney was winding down his career at Braintree Children's, working a holiday shift on a slow Thanksgiving afternoon when he heard the car come to a screeching halt.

A nurse was outside having a cigarette since the hospital itself had become a non-smoking building. She helped the couple carry the unresponsive, five-year-old child into the emergency room.

All other items of business were dropped as CODE BLUE was called over the hospital paging system. The EKG technician dropped what she was doing and rushed, the respiratory therapist on the third floor rushed, the charge nurse in the ICU rushed as they heard, "PEDIATRIC CODE BLUE" over the loudspeaker. They all stopped for less than a second wondering where their own children were at that moment. They ran down the stairs since no one waited for the elevator when CODE BLUE was called, especially PEDIATRIC CODE BLUE. Then they heard over the loudspeaker system, "WOULD ANY PEDIATRICIAN IN THE HOSPITAL PLEASE COME DOWN TO THE EMERGENCY ROOM RIGHT AWAY," and their hearts stopped for less than a second while they counted their own children one more time trying to place their whereabouts, and what they might be doing at that exact moment.

The procedurally-skilled Mahoney first placed a breathing tube into the cyanotic child's trachea to ventilate her with oxygen, a very efficient modality of resuscitation, and indeed, she pinked up a bit.

What wasn't so efficient was trying to speed up her slowing heart rate. Her heart rate should have been about one hundred beats per minute, but had now slowed to twenty-four beats per minute.

Mahoney first gave the intravenous solution of glucose, then ordered via protocol the narcotic antidote Narcan. He ascertained from the family the child was autistic, but had no history of other congenital diseases. He proceeded with attempts to speed up her heart rate with pharmacologic agents, but to no avail. The suction machine, of course, initially failed, and things seemed to be moving too slowly, nothing making a well-oiled, community-hospital's emergency department come unglued quicker than a pediatric arrest.

Mahoney was able to apply the transcutaneous pacemaker which did raise the child's heart rate, stabilizing her blood pressure as well. She became somewhat responsive, but before she fully awakened, Mahoney quickly and deftly slid a large tube into her stomach to empty it (pump her stomach), still thinking of the possibility of an ingestion, especially in an autistic child.

When he put down the large-bore, garden hose of a tube through her mouth into her gut, he quickly retrieved a literal basket of green leaves, everyone staring at the harvest.

The girl's father said, "I recently planted some ornamental shrubs in the front yard, but I don't know what they are."

Mahoney remembered that one of the patients waiting for an x-ray of his ankle was a landscaper, and Mahoney took some of the larger specimens for him to examine.

The landscaper said, "Without doubt, they're yew leaves, a

common shrub often used in my designs."

Mahoney called Massachusetts Poison Control, and the excellent group told Mahoney that yew leaves possessed a digitalis-like substance, and the girl was digitalis toxic, which readily explained the slowing of her heart rate.

Mahoney ordered the recently-developed antibodies to digitalis which cross reacted with the analogues in the yew leaves, and the girl's recovery was rapid, almost miraculous. The child did well as the pediatrician came in, without first asking the insurance status of the child. Mahoney's shift ended, and the baton was passed to his replacement, a moonlighting resident.

Three recent developments saved the child's life. The first was the transcutaneous pacemaker which simply required the placement of two large, sticky, pancake-like leads on the chest and back. Before its development, the only way to insert a pacemaker to the heart was through a large catheter threaded through a major vein, major veins notoriously difficult to cannulate in a child, especially a hypotensive one.

The new digitalis antibodies were a strikingly-effective development, changing dig-toxicity from a nightmarish complication to an easily treated entity.

The third recent development was the formal, emergency medicine training programs of specialty physicians dealing with life-threatening emergencies in high-risk patients from pediatrics to geriatrics, taking all of medicine a long way from the white-to-black Cadillac transition.

The total bill for the child's resuscitation was eight hundred dollars. Four hundred went to the hospital, three hundred and fifty dollars went to Goldman, and fifty dollars went to Mahoney.

Tahoe and their daughter arrived early to pick up Mahoney from work. They were going to have Thanksgiving dinner at Doctor Steinerman's house, the Steinerman family holding court at six p.m.

Mahoney told Tahoe the whole story in an animated fashion, excited because it was such a good save, but Tahoe, who'd arrived at the hospital thirty minutes early, had a little story of her own to tell.

It was four thirty when the moonlighting ophthalmology resident from Boston, who was to relieve Mahoney drove up and parked.

Tahoe was touched by the fact he'd come in early to relieve Mahoney on the holiday. As the moonlighting resident was getting out of his car, the family with the autistic child drove up beeping their horn, shouting, unloading a literally blue girl, obviously in a full respiratory arrest. The smoking nurse gave the child one Heimlich thrust, and three quick mouth-to-mouth breaths while the parents held her, and then rushed her into the emergency room.

Out of the corner of her eye, Tahoe saw with disbelief the resident, who was about to relieve Mahoney early, step back into his car, looking at his watch, not so anxious any more to do Mahoney a favor by coming on early, certainly not in light of this. She watched the resident dutifully look at his watch, going in at exactly thirty seconds to five o'clock, not realizing he was being watched by Tahoe.

But one shouldn't be the first to cast stones on this poor, moonlighting boy because most doctors, outside of emergency physicians and pediatricians, never see five-year olds in distress, let alone in a full respiratory arrest.

Many nail-biting, Maalox-munching residents are fully aware they are in over their heads the first day they are shot out of the cannon to fly solo in an emergency room outside of the University Hospital.

They certainly know enough not to immerse themselves into a quagmire, especially if there's the potential of relieving one of Lyle's **P**ontius **P**ilate **P**rofessors, someone who might quickly wash their hands of the matter, leaving the child's blood on their hands. No new eye surgeon wants to shoot his brilliant career in the foot this way. Tahoe was simply getting a little glimpse from the book of Revelations, emergency medicine style, and when she finished her story, the shocked Mahoney stared in disbelief.

Steinerman, Eileen, and Annie arrived first at the Steinerman household for the holiday dinner. While everyone exchanged pleasantries, Doctor and Steinerman immediately began their ritualistic disagreement on some aspect of medical care. The debate never began until Doctor's first born arrived, Doctor Steinerman knowing exactly the right buttons to push.

"I don't think the younger physicians are using enough antibiotics. Eileen and you don't remember the days when we had entire hospitals with nothing but kids with rheumatic fever from untreated strep throats. They're accusing us old timers today of the indiscriminate use of antibiotics, but think about it, we wiped out rheumatic fever, those horrible draining mastoid infections you don't see anymore, and the bronchiectasis you kids only read about today in *Harrison's* textbook."

"That's not true dad," Steinerman picking up immediately, "there's too much overuse of antibiotics by everyone today. All it does is cause organisms to mutate into much more resistant strains, and then we need more and newer antibiotics to treat the organisms we've created. Look at what's happening in the burn units."

"That's only in the hospital, Abe. There are no resistant strep bugs in the community and that's because..." but Doctor was interrupted by the door bell which signaled the end of the match until Steinerman's next visit.

Eileen had visited the Steinermans several times, and all in all, she did agree with Doctor Steinerman on two occasions, and had one split decision. This was no old fool speaking, but a thinker, although a contrarian thinker, never saying anything he hadn't reviewed in his cerebrum at some length.

Uncle Herschel, Doctor Steinerman's brother, had just arrived from New York City along with aunts, cousins, and seconds removed of each. Uncle Herschel was unmitigatedly joyous to see his favorite nephew Abe, and was ecstatic with the gloriously beautiful Eileen Chen, diving into the conversation, yacking as hard as he could at the brilliant Steinerman and Eileen.

Doctor Steinerman presided over the day, maintaining a small element of crowd control.

Uncle Herschel rose with obvious apprehension when Philip Mahoney and Tahoe, child in tow, entered the celebration. Uncle Herschel had used his Massachusetts Bar quite often during Philip Mahoney's adolescence, actually studying for the Pennsylvania Bar when Mahoney was admitted to the now defunct Hershey Medical School's emergency medicine residency program. Mahoney was not a troubled youth, simply a very troublesome youth. Uncle Herschel greeted the prodigal Mahoney by the hand as the grateful Philip, full of remembrances of misdemeanors past, hugged his "Uncle Herschel," introducing him proudly to Tahoe and their new baby. Uncle Herschel saw the felonious look in the baby's blue-green eyes recombinated from the genomes of their wild at heart parents, and wondered about buying some books on juvenile law.

There was a short, a very short, remembrance of Grandfather Steinerman before dinner began. Grandfather Steinerman had always begun holiday dinners with the question to Doctor Steinerman and Steinerman, "What about the knife? What about the knife?"

The group of head-bowed internists had to sit there in apology for not being surgeons while Uncle Hershel snickered. But now Grandfather was gone and the family gave thanks.

The meal commenced, and Uncle Hershel became quite confused at his nephew's mastery of contract law. He bantered back and forth, but Abraham seemed to know the distinctions of offers, consideration, and restrictive covenants. He looked at the deceptively bright Mahoney, but found him completely befuddled as to the basics of contract law or any other aspect of law.

Where did Abraham learn all of this? Uncle Herschel had wanted Steinerman to go to law school, but Steinerman never had the inclination. Had he been attending night school on the sly? He turned to Eileen who had the obvious aptitude, but again, no inclination and certainly no mastery of even the basics.

He quizzed Abe, "Where the hell have you been studying all this anyway?"

Steinerman explained, "I just got back from a series of meetings sponsored by the American Academy of Emergency Physicians."

"The American Academy of Emergency Physicians? Well," said Uncle Herschel, "I just went to a meeting of the New York Bar Association, but I don't remember any lectures on congenital heart disease."

Steinerman looked at Philip, Tahoe and Eileen. He then looked at his aunts, cousins, and father while everyone looked for an explanation. Steinerman was looking for an answer. Everyone stopped eating, waiting. Had Steinerman indeed been secretly attending law school? Steinerman groped. Then it suddenly came to him. "That is the answer! The meetings of the Academy! I've been attending the officially-sponsored meetings of the American Academy for the past year, and that's where I've picked up all this law, especially contract law."

What no one had realized was that the American Academy of Emergency Physicians had a certain de-emphasis on thrombolysis, croup, trichomonas, meningitis and prehospital care. The national meetings centered on quality assurance, market diversification, torts, the crises of the nonexistent malpractice crises, and above all, the noncompete clause.

Steinerman muddled on, speaking of various forms of risk management, and a somewhat confused theory of negligence. "I started splinting all injured wrists just in case they might be fractured. That fulfills my duty of care to the patient. If the patient removes the splint, the patient would then have contributed to his own negligence if the wrist was indeed fractured. Blind splinting allows time for the radiologist to overread the x-ray the next day if I misread the film. I can then call the patient, fulfilling my duty of follow-up, and won't be the proximate cause of any damages the patient might sustain afterwards. I also..."

"O.k, o.k., o.k., Abe," said Uncle Hershel, studying his own wrist, getting a little hot under the collar. "Abe, why don't you just learn how to read the x-rays? Surely the American Academy must have meetings on that?" Steinerman wasn't quite clicking, but sensed Uncle Hershel was right.

Eileen was somewhat stunned as well, turning to Steinerman, "You know, darling, I could teach you in a few afternoons." It certainly struck Eileen as bizarre that Steinerman would defensively splint every wrist he x-rayed, especially since everyone knew most of the wrists didn't really need an x-ray in the first place.

Eileen added, "It does seem like a roundabout way to do things, to practice medicine, and do this risk-management thing. Besides, those splints are pretty uncomfortable."

Then Steinerman corrected her, "No, honey, it's not risk management, it's quality assurance. Risk management comes after the..."

"Risk against what, the child developing a worse injury?" snapped Eileen, her patience wearing thin at all this claptrap.

"Well, no," said Steinerman, "It's quality assurance against being successfully sued." The chart-wars mentality began to afflict the normally clear-thinking Steinerman.

Everyone sensed the inexplicable, illogic of this topsy-turvy reasoning, but the Tower of Babel Steinerman continued to babble on, misusing words and expressions like "duty," "the prudent physician," "due diligence," and hospitals can't "run and hide," while Uncle Hershel became hotter and hotter, finally having a mini-explosion when Steinerman said "res ipsa loquitor."

The dinner conversation suddenly changed, since the entire family was bored by all this Greek, and they began exchanging stories, gossip, and inquiring-mind stuff, things everyone really wanted to discuss.

Steinerman withdrew and became melancholic, thinking of Nightingale, his wife and their two children, a fatherless family he could have prevented. He thought of the melancholy of their holiday, their certain void, emptiness. He looked at Mahoney, busy eating, and remembered Mahoney had told him emergency medicine was different. It wasn't so much the inevitable or the old, but the young vibrant ectopics one lost, fathers and mothers that one didn't click on one night, kids orphaned by the simple misreading of a cardiogram. "You remember them on holidays by name," Mahoney had told him, "not just as infarcts or ectopics, not only by Death & Doughnuts, but on a holiday by face and name, and a simple thought of what you might have done." Steinerman felt ever so guilty. Ironically, he not only didn't fear a malpractice suit, but welcomed it. Certainly a simple guilty plea would expiate this feeling Mahoney warned would be recurrent, the ceaseless self-interrogation about a death he could have prevented. "It was just a fuck up," he could say, and tell his Bahamian Island insurance company to pay up. But Mrs. Nightingale hadn't sued, and suddenly he came to a conclusion at which even the omniscient Mahoney hadn't arrived—America wasn't such a litigious society! Most people don't sue even when they have cause. It was indeed a hoax, and he felt like calling Mrs. Nightingale. "Sue me! I have insurance! Sue me. It's just a few hundred thou out of Grand Bahamian, Inc." Sue and forgive? Maybe, maybe not.

After dinner Uncle Hershel sat everyone down and gave a small history lesson.

"When I was in law school, one of my favorite courses was a fall semester in my third year in medical malpractice taught by a practicing cardiologist who also had a law degree. The doctor-patient relationship used to be viewed by the courts as a contract between two people, but the law soon realized the relationship was not a simple contract. If the patient was wronged because of the doctor, the law had to provide an adequate remedy. So malpractice was no longer a subject in the books of contract law, but moved to the textbook of tort law, now found in the chapters on negligence.

"In the old days, doctors had powerful state and county medical societies, and all the doctors participated in what was called the 'conspiracy of silence,' never testifying against another doctor regardless of what the accused did.

"In all courts in the United States today, malpractice cases require expert witnesses, the courts recognizing only physicians as expert witnesses, and not nurses, public-health officials, optometrists, dentists, chiropractors, Ph.D.s, psychologists, pharmacists or podiatrists. Only M.D. and osteopathic physicians are court-approved expert witnesses.

"If plaintiffs couldn't find a physician willing to testify in their behalf, the case was dropped, and many, many valid cases were simply dropped in the old days. The lawyers then got pretty creative.

"I remember the landmark case involving a lady who went in for an amputation of her left leg, but instead, because of a 'clerical error,' she got her right leg amputated below the knee. She sued, but couldn't find a physician willing to break the conspiracy of silence. Her attorney changed the action from a malpractice or negligence issue to a consent issue, saying the woman never consented to have the good leg cut off. The courts agreed, awarding her damages, and since it was a consent case, and not a malpractice case, the courts didn't require an expert witness.

"This is the reason why this so called 'informed consent' is such an overblown issue today, certainly something you boys in the emergency room should never worry about. There has never been a successful consent action won by a plaintiff against a physician for taking emergency action that has ever been upheld by the appeals courts. This simply makes good public-policy sense. The appellate court is well aware they don't want to provide a disincentive to any physician, anywhere, even within the hospital, for taking emergency actions.

So always remember to err on the side of treatment of the patient. A twelve-membered jury will forgive the so-called 'four D's'—the dumb, dedicated, documented doctor. They're not likely to forgive some doctor who thinks he's a legal beagle, withholding treatment on a literal technicality.

"Of course in today's society, the conspiracy of silence has long since ended. One can see in any legal journal scores of companies offering physicians to testify in medical-malpractice cases. In fact, many of your rapscallion 'suits' were amongst the first to break ranks. There's actually a glut of expert witnesses today, ready and willing, if not fully able, to testify against other doctors.

"Remember, not all cases are meritless. One of the cases we had in class involved a woman who appeared in the emergency room at three a.m. wanting a diet. The emergency physician was asleep, and told the nurses to give her a diet, went back to sleep, and saw the woman four hours later, but this time in a full cardiac arrest.

"You boys and ladies know this better than I, but apparently the woman was in congestive heart failure. Because she couldn't pump blood through her vessels adequately, she accumulated fluid in her extremities. This edema in her legs became massive, elephantine, and she gained fifty pounds. She came in at three a.m. because when she lay down, the fluid redistributed into her lungs, and the shortness of breath woke her up. She then came to the emergency room.

"If the doctor on call hadn't said, 'Oh, crap on it,' and had seen her, he would have given her the so-called 'last clear chance,' and the diet of diuretics and digitalis which she needed. Instead she was sent home to drown in her own bed in her own fluids (the 'go home and drown in your own fluids' patient). So he indeed breached his duty to the patient.

"One of his defenses was that he hadn't established a doctor- patient relationship with the woman, but the court said as soon as she strolled through the doors of the hospital, the relationship was established. Emergency department physicians are not allowed to choose which patients they will see."

"Why didn't they sue the nurse?" Tahoe asked.

"Because," Uncle Hershel continued, "even though the nurse was in the wrong, just wanting to get back to the coffee lounge herself, she only had ten thousand dollars worth of malpractice insurance. The doctor had the 'deep pocket.' His million-dollar insurance policy was the one the plaintiff's attorney wanted."

"Well, in those cases, I guess it was beyond a reasonable doubt they were guilty," said Mahoney.

Uncle Hershel was again astonished at the ignorance of physicians regarding even the most fundamental principles of law, saying, "Philip, I've told you repeatedly in the past, civil cases are decided by a 'preponderance of the evidence,' fifty-one per cent of the tilt, and not by the heavier weight of 'beyond a reasonable doubt.'

"Yes, of course, society wants the evidence to be beyond a reasonable doubt before sending someone to the electric chair, but the evidence has only to be 'more likely than not' to convict an individual in the civil action of negligence.

"One of the most dangerous things you doctors do, and do regularly, is maintain your illiteracy in the law. Do you realize all attorneys in the United States of America know that there are seven cervical vertebral bodies, and yet physicians can't even distinguish between the civil and the criminal law? It's almost contemptuous, Doctors."

"Tell us another case," Eileen pleaded.

"Well, for some reason this is one of my favorites. We went over a case involving a psychiatrist who was confronted by a patient with a gun. The two of them were alone in the doctor's office when the patient told the psychiatrist he had homicidal ideations and wanted to kill someone, anyone. The psychiatrist conducted the interview with complete imperturbability, even though the gun was pointed straight at him, until about thirty minutes into the session when the patient agreed with the therapist that he had lost his homicidal feelings, and handed his gun over to the shrink. The shrink continued the session, and when the timer buzzed, signaling the end of the forty-five minute session, the psychiatrist, believe it or not, gave the patient back his gun. The patient went out," while Uncle Hershel waited a minute for the uproarious laughter to abate, "the patient went out to the bathroom and shot himself," which made everyone in the room howl even louder. "The family sued the shrink...,

"Well that one's beyond a reasonable doubt," shouted Mahoney.

"Wrong again, Philip. A conservative Southern jury said the entire event was unforeseeable," causing an immediate standing ovation by all, no one quite certain if the joyous applause was due to Philip Mahoney's being wrong again or because the doctor beat the rap.

Uncle Hershel then changed the subject, saying to Steinerman, "Elaborate more for me on this pork-barrel 'management' and other aspects of emergency medicine mountebankery."

As he listened, he became visibly perturbed, and what Uncle Hershel seemed to hate the most was market diversification, that's what disturbed him the most, the well-padded market diversification.

"Criminal lawyers, product-liability lawyers, divorce lawyers, and bankruptcy lawyers don't diversify, but now you're telling me about hair transplants?" asked the startled Uncle Hershel.

"You're telling me the American Academy of Emergency Physicians is sponsoring meetings suggesting idle doctors in the 'doc in the boxes' learn how to perform hair transplants in their spare time? Between cardiac arrests and the Swine flu, these doctors Monk and Walsh can transplant tufts of hair? This is the official direction and advice of the American Academy?"

The horror hit Uncle Hershel. "My God," he said, "children are not safe under the Goldman or Pinnacle, Inc., plan. I'm in a fair amount of danger myself under the sexual-restraint plan of Pyramid. What this specialty really needs is de-diversification. Why do you boys belong to the Academy anyway?"

But neither had an answer. Steinerman and Mahoney (along with eleven thousand other very fine physicians) simply stated they belonged to the organization without ever explaining why.

Uncle Hershel replied, "I don't belong to non-obligatory clubs, especially ones that would have me so easily as a member."

Doctor Steinerman chimed in with, "I do belong to the American College of Rheumatology because it doesn't advise doing hair transplants, nor does it have crips, bloods, weasels, Rolodexes, mosquitoes, sidekicks, war rooms, green pins, yellow pins that change to red pins, state secrets called proprietary information, pledge drivers, or thumbs up their asses, although it certainly does have its share of heads in the ozone academics. Also, it doesn't hire Rheumatologists in a nationwide, centralized plan to go out and see the crippled patients, and then send 'management' residuals to the 'suit' who established the beachhead first."

Philip Mahoney then told Uncle Hershel the whole story. Steinerman mentioned it was Goldman who'd given the lecture on contracts, publicly claiming he was losing money on Braintree Children's, but decided for the good of emergency medicine everywhere to enforce the noncompete clause which Uncle Hershel had instinctively known at this point was unenforceable.

"In other words, it sounds like economic intimidation by the larger army," said Uncle Hershel. "They know they can't win, but can tie you up in the courts long enough to steer you into the financial shoals. They know damn well they can't prevail in a court of law! But they sure can shut you up for the time being with the specter of prolonged, complicated, and costly litigation. It's a simple vendetta, and a well-known ploy of well-heeled companies to fight their critics, usually the honest critics. These lawsuits are known within the legal community as 'intimidation suits,' designed to punish people in a war of attrition, making everyone think twice about speaking out against the empire.

"I can see where it would be an especially effective stratagem against a recently-graduated physician with a new house and young family. Is that what the leadership is saying they'll do to you? And this is all done against their own people? What the hell kind of an organization is this, anyway?"

Uncle Hershel had forgotten how far removed the general population is from the law. "This contract malarkey they're trying to use as a battering ram against decency might be the letter of the law, but not the spirit. It's certainly not the interpretation Oliver Wendell Holmes or Justice Brandeis might give it. You guys are doctors, seeing patients, and the spirit of the law doesn't restrain from good medical care." He was furious with Mahoney for not coming to him sooner.

Uncle Hershel listened more closely to the cheap, petty, sordid, mean-spirited, spoil-sport thing that was happening to Philip Mahoney in the name of a medical specialty with their own unholy alliance with the law, and he did something that no one in the family outside of Doctor had ever seen before.

Doctor Steinerman remembered it from a long time ago when he was twelve years old and had borrowed, without authorization, Uncle Hershel's baseball glove. Uncle Hershel became completely glandular, his face reddened, sweat poured out, and all of a sudden he flew into a rage. The family was stunned, but it was refreshing for Doctor to see his brother as his old self. "My," Doctor Steinerman declared as he watched his brother rant and rave, "how we've become civilized."

All in all, it was a wonderful and memorable holiday for everyone. Early the next day Mahoney and Steinerman saw Uncle Hershel and the family off, and both Mahoney and Steinerman went to join many of the medical families of Boston for the great festive event that morning. It was time for everyone to rush over to Boston University's Death and Doughnuts conference, now Bagels, Cream Cheese, Death and Doughnuts.

Everyone knew it would be crowded because Sheila Schultz's ovaries were on the chopping block. Dr. S. Schultz had managed to piss off everyone in Boston and beyond, and therefore, a big, hostile crowd was expected. By eight a.m. a carnival-like atmosphere developed, and the pathology department had to send off for more delicious doughnuts.

Riley was the visiting surgeon from Indiana in charge of today's Death and Doughnuts, and to everyone's delight, Doctor Schultz would be sitting on the stool by herself for two cases: one a missed appendicitis; and the other a botched, abdominal gunshot wound.

The eminently distinguished statesman of surgery, the silver-haired Doctor Riley, read the first case, looking splendid in his long white coat. He delivered the reading of the first case like a man of letters, but wasn't quite prepared for Schultz, and before he could even finish, she snapped, "Why didn't the surgical resident who saw her first perform a rectal exam, or is that not part of the abdominal examination in Boston any more?"

Everyone watched Doctor Riley lower his right hand, reaching for his Louisville Slugger to knock the doughnut out of her hand and bash her brains out, but the yellow-bellied Indianian stopped, and suddenly admitted it was the surgical resident's fault, but not before Schultz quipped,

"Do they do rectals in Indiana, Doctor Riley, or is it still, 'when in doubt, cut it out?'"

Riley was stunned, but managed to begin reading the botched, gunshot-wound case when suddenly Schultz pulled back the big, black curtain behind her, revealing a huge, bright-yellow steamroller which she jumped onto, starting up its roaring engines. Riley could hardly be heard over the roar of the engines as she screamed, "I don't understand exactly what you're saying about our gunshot-wound statistics in Boston, Doctor Riley. Are you people in Indiana just better surgeons, or are our citizens in Boston better marksmen?"

Riley stood there holding his huge uneaten doughnut, knowing his published statistics were a bit sloppy, and many *fellows* cringed, remembering those ridiculous stats published in *The Journal of Trauma.*

Schultz put the six-ton monster on full throttle and flattened Riley right there in front of everyone. People coughed from the diesel fumes, and the male doctors in the front row threw their hands up to avoid being splattered with the raspberry filling. The males were furious while the vicious Schultz kept gleefully juggling with the controls, backing over Riley, who muttered something about sewing the omentum over the liver in bad cases, but it only annoyed her more. She blew the whistle on the big yellow steamroller, letting it rip, "That's frosting on the cake and you know it. The trauma surgeons don't waste their time on that here in Boston," as she kept it up, back and forth, back and forth and O, *the horror, the horror* as Riley kept getting flatter and flatter.

A group of about fifteen orthopedists in the upper, left-hand corner of the auditorium was steamin', but they noticed fifty-one per cent of the new physicians in Boston were now women. Eileen Chen's presence in the lower, right-hand corner did not go unnoticed either.

Suddenly the awful odor of hot roofing tar permeated the air, and no one believed that fucking ruthless bitch would do it, but Riley screeched as the black liquid poured all over him, feeling worse than a hot sugar burn. Schultz sprinkled the feathers on him as he retracted his data saying he was sorry he published those stats in *The Journal of Trauma.* Everyone had to listen to that horribly malicious, diabolical laugh of Sheila Schultz's as she sat there, high up on the steamroller, telling Riley to go back to Indiana and sin no more.

Although the males were too scared at the moment to do anything, a Robert Bly-like bonding developed, especially when Schultz started impugning Riley's father, and they just couldn't stand it any longer, seeing Riley flattened like a victim of one of Goldman's soda machines with jelly smeared all over his gleaming white coat, and then tarred over like the Massachusetts Turnpike and chicken feathered, but no one could help him now. Afterwards, all the New England male doctors got together, resoundingly denying the whole incident had ever happened, and had that morning's seminar deleted from the Annals of Death and Doughnuts.

Because the deleted event went into overtime, Steinerman was late for his day shift at St. Joseph's Hospital, but it turned out to be an easy day in the emergency department.

After discharging his last patient late in the afternoon, and while waiting for Monk to relieve him, he strolled over to the radiology suite to see Eileen, just after the janitors had finished waxing the floors, when he suddenly slipped and fell in the radiology department. They all heard the crack as this freak occurrence snapped his femur like a dry twig. They put him on a stretcher, and wheeled him onto the x-ray table.

Eileen read the film, and told him it looked like surgery, but he was in such a state of disbelief, the pain didn't quite hit. The shift was nearly over, and Monk relieved him while Steinerman directed his own preliminary care, almost laughing in shock at this silly event. Eileen was sitting with Steinerman when Monk came over, sincerely asking if their was anything he could do.

Steinerman, now aware of the pain, and in a rare moment of sarcasm, said, "Yeah, get me a Big Mac in a box, doc." Monk missed it.

Eileen was very distressed, full of remorse over Steinerman's fall, but since her undeserved guilt wasn't helping anyone, she leaned over, kissed him on the lips, and called the large Cat a clumsy oaf. She also glanced at Monk, whispering to Steinerman, "I think that man has a Valium-secreting tumor." Steinerman laughed until it literally hurt.

Monk left, but reappeared fifteen minutes later. He'd sent the orderly out on an errand, and had a McDonald's bag in his hand, a Big Mac for the Cat. How touching, even Steinerman had to think. Of course, Steinerman was going to emergency surgery, and could have no food or water by mouth because one of the most common causes of death is aspiration, just like the John Fay case.

Eileen thanked Monk, told him not to worry since the orthopedist would be in shortly, and took the hamburger away from Steinerman who in his pain and hunger had forgotten the upcoming procedure. Too bad he didn't have an undiagnosed ruptured spleen—Monk would have been more generous with the morphine.

Where was Westerly when you needed him? Monk as usual was not actively, but passively homicidal, like a bridge for the unwary motorist that had been washed away in a storm.

Steinerman went to the operating room thinking of the Big Mac filling his trachea and right-main-stem bronchial tube, shutting off an entire lung. Thank God, anesthesia, surgery, and orthopedics weren't run like franchised emergency rooms or he'd be a goner for sure. He thought he might die anyway, but it was a strangely pleasant thought. Drifting off under the induction of anesthesia, he had a dream-like, near-death experience, but it wasn't the white, brilliantly-lighted tunnel everyone spoke about. When the Pentathol hit, there he was, dancing rather blissfully with Eileen, waltzing through the Golden Arches.

CHAPTER TWENTY-THREE

THE THOUSAND YEAR PYRAMID

"The practice of medicine is an art, not a trade; a calling, not a business."
—*Sir William Osler, M.D.*

Old Osler could have learned a thing or two from Lyle and Goldman.

Lyle was presently winding down his latest European trip. His fondness for the old civilizations grew each year, and he felt he truly fit into the European schema, especially the English-speaking part.

He always took an early morning walk through London on Harley Street, a street made famous throughout the centuries by the offices of world-famous English physicians, doctors who received referrals from the Sheiks of Saudi and the Crown Princes of Thailand.

As a child, Lyle had always loved reading English history while staring in envy at the cupolas of Francis Peabody's home, where he now maintained his Boston residence.

He'd read where the physicians of Harley Street banded together in the late eighteen hundreds to prevent dermatologists from renting offices on the famous street because so many of the dermatology patients had such grotesque rashes. The urologists and surgeons didn't want their own patients to see the disfigurement, lest the patients feel the doctors of

Harley Street weren't such great therapists after all. It was simply bad publicity, and Lyle hated bad publicity. The interdiction of dermatologists on Harley Street was a good marketing move, and Lyle loved good marketing moves.

Whenever in London, Norman always looked on Harley Street for vacant offices or buildings for sale. It was his dream to own an historical English townhouse, and put a kitchen scheduling office there, a satellite representing his new international consulting firm to provide global emergency medicine leadership. The time had come to introduce his very own "Massachusetts Plan" on the steps of Westminster, to privatize the emergency rooms of the Commonwealth. France could be next, expanding the theater of operations along the worldwide *Rue des Pyramides*. Surely the local physicians could have no objection to that?

Lyle strolled back to his Bed and Breakfast suite after picking up some mail from the Colonies. He'd just gotten the results of the questionnaire he'd authorized for the study of patient response to the care in his "managed" emergency rooms. Lyle actually deserved a little credit for putting out the questionnaire, asking the public to reflect on his collection of Monks and Walshes.

He was quite apprehensive, expecting some heavy fallout from the results of the questionnaire, a rather detailed one given out to patients and their families leaving the emergency room. Lyle knew the patients were like the "scrubs," nothing but trouble, wishing there would be some way in the future to run a utopian emergency room without patients or "scrubs."

He got a forty-percent return rate on the questionnaire, and expected to take quite a drubbing on the generics. Before opening the responses, Lyle closed his eyes tightly, whispering, "God save the Queen."

But to his utter surprise, most of the really sick patients didn't have complaints about the doctors, any complaints at all. The cardiacs, the bleeders, and the families of the automobile crunch victims had only good things to say. It was the toenails, the worried well, the walking wounded who bitched the loudest.

And what did they complain about? The long waiting time before they got to see a doctor was their primary complaint, but running a close second was the proximity of the vending machines. Slow physician response time and the lack of an express check-in counter were understandable, but the proximity of the coffee machine to the waiting area? The patients said they had to walk too far to get a Pepsi or a some Twinkies. Also, the television in the cinderblock-walled waiting room didn't get enough channels.

The patients from the suburbs of Boston were middle-class, medically-insured, blue-collar folks who graduated from one of Boston's seventeen public schools, but even those who went to the Latin, with its revised requirements because of the perceived black threat, were still not quite the brie-and-chablis set.

A few respondents groused about the Gestapo-like clerk who fully depersonalized them by demanding insurance information, and asking unanswerable questions analogous to "What is the meaning of life?"

There were a few complaints about the cheap, plastic chairs on which they had to sit, and the herd-like roundup of the waiting room, but most astonishingly, there were very few complaints about the doctors themselves. The vast majority didn't know the difference between a Monk or a Steinerman. The strep throats and sprained ankles came to the hospital's billboard-advertised emergency department, their only complaint being not enough bread and circuses.

It puzzled Lyle, and he suddenly remembered Goldman. Goldman must have realized this long ago, and that's why he bought those soda machines, taking pains to make sure the machines were properly bolted to the floor so the brats wouldn't tip them over, get crushed, and have to be sent to a Level One Trauma Center in the Econolines, even if they got crushed in the waiting room of a Level Two hospital. How perceptive of

Goldman, Lyle thought.

Norman and Carolyn stayed at the very same Bed and Breakfast every time they came to London, from the time he'd thought of the loss leader and the endowed chair of emergency medicine, until now. It was in the idleness of the British Empire where Lyle usually concocted new schemes to broaden the base of the Pyramid. He liked the privacy of the study, and enjoyed the Benedictine and Brandy, his nightly grand indulgence when traveling.

Their suite had a small private library attached to their bedroom, a "quiet room," but not of the sort that had caused so much trouble in gastroenterology. The Elizabethan richness of the supremely-appointed library contained *objets d'art* sitting on elegant, elaborately-inlaid pedestals, resting on plush Persian carpets. The built-in, solid walnut bookcases were full of gold-leaf books and polished brass, looking over an oversized, glove-leather chair where Lyle sat alone, one of the few times in his life when he had the luxury to simply sit and think in solitude.

Norman Lyle was certainly not the type of individual given to introspection, but two things conspired this time for a review of his life and legacy. The previous sot who'd rented the Bed and Breakfast had broken all the cognac glasses, leaving only the much larger wine glasses. He wasn't used to the extra alcohol, and it made him uncharacteristically sentimental, tearful in spots.

More importantly, Lyle had heard that the ex-Hershey residents were planning an unauthorized biography of him and the Pyramid. He knew it was time to officially commission his magisterial biography, the real history of emergency medicine, a story in the true Shakespearean sense that needed to be told.

He began to reminisce the happy trails of his extraordinary past, looking at a few entries in his diary. He thought of emergency medicine and the kitchen where he and Carolyn began almost twenty years ago simply scheduling "scrubs," and how, at the time, he viewed kitchen scheduling as nothing more than a sophomoric excess, so afraid the authorities might find out about the five dollars an hour he skimmed off the unsuspecting plebes. But now kitchen scheduling had evolved to become "management" with a preordained fat cut of the action. It had gotten so much more complicated, the O-J-T-ers for example. He laughed, reading about the fat, stubby one who collapsed at lunch.

Lyle never could have imagined twenty years later, he and Carolyn would still be kitchen scheduling with silicon-circuitry Rolodexes, desktop-publishing glossies, salaried pledge drivers, commissioned mosquitoes, Bing and the "start-up-set-up" physicians followed by the old switcharoos, and a master corporate war room to fight the other crips and bloods. Surprisingly, they had even received honors and awards by a then-unknown organization, the American Academy of Emergency Physicians. Now he and Carolyn manipulated the Academy, funding award ceremonies so Pyramid, Inc., could do the giving instead of receiving.

As an afterthought, and a most disagreeable one, Lyle remembered those loosely strung marionettes, the "scrubs." He almost forgot about that set of sixty thousand extras who were also part of the story, none of them worth a farthing in his mind, noting there were no pleasant entries in the diary about them.

But Lyle was deeply bothered by something. He could never understand why Goldman was relatively well-liked by the "scrubs" and he wasn't. Goldman wasn't even a nice guy. He was the owner of a set of emergency room contracts as worthless as Pyramid's, some with even higher kill ratios. Lyle couldn't understand why he was singled out for the resentment of the "scrubs," for he never out and out lied to anyone.

"Well, shit," he suddenly realized, "this isn't cricket, it's just sour grapes on their part. They would have done the same thing I did if they'd had the sporting chance to be in my shoes." But still he seethed the way he used to at Doctor Peabody, becoming especially enraged when he remembered that small group of hooligans, those ex-residents from the ex-Hershey Med Center program who threw spitballs at the Pyramid, Inc., float in New Orleans during Kensington's Apollo moonshot speech. Like so many "suits," Lyle's rage autocatalytically escalated into a near social meltdown. He poured himself another generous B & B straight up into his capacious wine glass.

He realized that no one except for his ladyship Carolyn knew how hard he'd worked to achieve all this.

"Carolyn," he thought, "She's like the Queen Mother of emergency medicine with all the modesty of queens as well."

In the solemnity of his thinking, he knew that he and Carolyn, like the dancers of the Royal Ballet, lived only for their art, kitchen scheduling.

"All those nights in the beginning," Lyle remembered, "hour after hour on the sugar frosted flakes counter, writing on the backs of envelopes, calling every doc in creation to fill in a blank. All those goddamned, frustrating flunkies, and fucking Walsh, that perennial no-show. How many times did I get those frantic Friday night phone calls telling me that Walsh or some other flight risk hadn't shown up, calls from the O-J-T-ers threatening to replace me with Goldman. I'd have to drive over to that purgatory of the Friday night emergency room for a tour of duty of battlefield medicine with the (uninsured) knife-and-gun club, personally filling in a blank like a 'scrub' after a hard day of 'managing.' I could have stayed at that cushy job at sugar frosted flakes, but I took the risk, choosing to be one of the bold young leaders of emergency medicine.

"And what about all that law I had to learn and all those accounting principles. I really am the renaissance emergency physician," Lyle rhapsodized, realizing again emergency medicine "management" had been the only thing in his and Carolyn's lives for the past twenty years.

"And then there was the bad advice. Oh, my God," he said aloud, "the bad advice like buying the company jet instead of leasing it, and then that idiotic law firm that incorporated the hospital contracts under six hundred separate incomprehensible layers 'for protection.'

"Hiring that so-so law firm was an extremely costly mistake, eventually costing (the 'scrubs') over a thousand dollars a year per contract just for franchise taxes.

"And that better-known law firm, with their proportionately immense fee, laughing at all the strategic planning, saying, 'Doctor Lyle, that's just hogwash. Any good attorney can pierce these corporate veils lickety-split. You need to dissolve these elaborate holding companies and corporations within corporations within corporations. Just get business insurance and form trust funds to park your assets beyond the reach of creditors, litigants, and regulators.'"

Lyle turned his anger to the "scrubs," those pirates who wanted to de-couple from the Pyramid's "management," pushing him back to the edge, but Lyle knew that just wasn't going to happen.

The "scrubs" had forgotten the original goal of the House of Lyle to Pyramidize the nation's emergency rooms—yes, a thousand emergency rooms to "manage" for a thousand years, an institution living on like the Royal Family of England, financed by its subjects, the serflike "scrubs," who would pay due royalties to Lyle and his blood line, for Norman J. Lyle was no interloper in emergency medicine, and wasn't going to "go gently into that dark night."

"Oh, they will know, and they will know in my lifetime," Lyle having that willingness-to-serve mentality crop up again, wondering what to say to the President when the President finally realized what it was the nation really needed—an emergency medicine Czar and his Czarina. He saw some loose coins on the dresser, realizing it was time they replaced Monticello on the reverse side of the nickel, replaced it with the Logo of the Pyramid, Inc. As his head turned slightly, he caught his own visage en profile in the mirror realizing how small he'd been thinking again. "It was me, and not Goldman, who singlehandedly founded the twenty-third formally recognized medical specialty. I am its single biggest icon. What about the front of the nickel?"

But the question of Goldman and his popularity kept going through his head. "How come Goldman fits and I don't? Never mind that," and pouring another glass, he realized he did fit, he fit into the ambitious nineteen-eighties, he was a businessman, a takeover artist, a shrewd player in a big game. As the rich vapors from the Benedictine & Brandy burned his nostrils, he realized he was, after all, the quintessence of his time, he was an entrepreneur. He remembered his apparition in the Hancock Building, the day he showed Mahoney and Steinerman the war room, how he saw God, and God was so well pleased with his beloved son Norman, his son the entrepreneur, the good thief. But like the bad thief, Lyle chuckled, "No matter how bad the doctors are, Pyramid still limits the death rate to one per patient."

Suddenly he busted out laughing, "The more I think like P.T. Barnum, the more successful I become."

Now the patients themselves had given the ringmaster of the emergency medicine "management" circus a whole new revelation in their own handwriting. There they were, between the "doc in the box" absurdities and his emergency rooms, receiving the worst possible medical care the nation had to offer, and what were they so irate about? Third-class waiting rooms without their Twinkies or MTV.

CHAPTER TWENTY-FOUR

NIGHTTIME

"The best way to rob a bank is to own one."
—*Old banking proverb*

During Steinerman's six-month recovery from a badly broken leg, he read and studied extensively, realized great Chinese cooking never kept any man thin, and sex without birth control makes a woman pregnant. He raised, with immense joy, his adopted daughter, Eileen's gorgeous little girl, Annie Thieu Yen Chen Steinerman.

He painstakingly acquired as much data as he could on the staggering amounts of money which the "management" groups and weasels were taking in. It was the happiest he'd been since the early days with Shelly. He'd get up with Eileen, have coffee, and then read for two hours. He'd get on the phone acquiring additional data from groups, doctors, billing services, and insurance companies, verifying astronomical figures time and time again. He would then pick Annie up at daycare, his working day done. Today Annie told him she wanted either a Jewish sister or a Chinese brother.

Steinerman loved the everydayness of his new life, living with Eileen and Annie, studying and researching the largest covert health care swindle in the history of American medicine. The scam was a combination of brilliant and creative marketing, expert salesmanship, and hit-and-miss doctors, all "managed" by a set of sociopathic, non-physician M.D.s armed with a catalogue of screwball "products" and "services."

Its elucidation was no small task, requiring a prodigious amount of detective work. He sleuthed around billing and malpractice companies looking for a way to strip-search the lying "suits." He got Dan Anderson to send him all the glossies he received from the crips and the bloods, but he got his biggest help from other emergency physicians.

There were many "scrubs" quite willing to name the fantastically rich crips, bloods, and weasels in their city, three in San Francisco, fifteen in greater L.A., two in San Diego, five in Dallas, eight in Houston, three in Jacksonville, and twenty in the very Fertile Crescent of the Greater Chicago Region.

As the list went on, Steinerman saw where these men neither created wealth nor provided real services, but siphoned monies off of fees originally intended for the hands-on doctors actually "caring for the patient." The only clever way to rob the emergency department was to own its contract, converting the clinical dollars into "management" money.

Steinerman saw the desperate hunger of the secessionist-minded "scrubs" to be freed from the shackles of the crips, and pry loose the boa-constrictor squeeze of the bloods. He heard many horror stories of the actions of the "suits" to maintain their "management" gravy trains, trains without brakemen. He began to see a group of seedy, underhanded misfits with no limits or set limitations scooping millions off the top.

The numbers of crips, bloods, and weasels grew, but as their numbers grew they began to shrink. Steinerman had long lists of names, but every time he added them up he saw less than two thousand names. He counted again, but the list shrank right in front of him now containing less than fifteen hundred names. There were close to twenty-five thousand "scrubs" in the country, but why less than fifteen hundred "suits?" Then it hit him. Many of the "suits" were ripping off several hospitals under the euphemism of "sound centralized management," and some of the crips and the bloods had a prodigious number of "management" contracts. Of course, each hospital needed five to ten "scrubs" to function, but still, less than fifteen hundred "suits?" No, wait a minute, could this be? It seemed like less than a thousand. Less than a thousand hustlers had destroyed a medical specialty over a twenty-year lost weekend? Could this be? "Yes, it's true," Steinerman gasped, remembering the New York City crack-cocaine-dealer line, "There's high dollars in it, Bro."

He also saw a several billion dollar figure that didn't change. "Oh, my God," he thought, "Mahoney and Anderson were way off base—several billion non-clinical dollars were distributed to less than one thousand 'suits.'"

Steinerman become frightened, seeing how this "honest graft" made literal fortunes with selected concentrations of wealth in emergency medicine's very own Fortune 500. He realized these men had split billions of kitchen scheduling dollars while the puppet regimes in the Academy closed their eyes. Steinerman was convinced the helpless Academy had no hope of cleaning its own house. It was too big a temptation, too much skimmed money in the parking meters for the "suits," too much at stake causing these men to so grievously breach the honor system, too much money leading to the falsifications and rampant lies—so much, so absolute, so irresistible, and so corrupting.

Steinerman had another revelation, another one of those damn passages of maturity when he suddenly realized he would have never come across this unless he had broken his leg. Unless he'd been laid up with a cast from his hip to his big toe, being taken care of by a good woman with a strong sense of family, and out of action from being a "scrub," he would have never investigated this so carefully.

In his entire life, he'd never once considered taking six months off from being a grunt in whatever it was—high-school achievement, college grade point, medical-school performance, internship, residency, and being a practitioner of emergency medicine—always a foot soldier on the front line all his life without ever decompressing. Like most new working doctors starting on the treadmill, he wasn't scheduled to come up for air for another thirty years. Never would he have taken six leisurely months off to investigate such a crime as emergency medicine "management." He'd always assumed someone else was doing it, someone else was looking into what was common knowledge. He then realized there was no police force of emergency medicine, no superego, he was the only one in the nation taking the time off to fully compile data estimating the magnitude of "a crime," the only person, even though everybody knew it was going on. No wonder they fired Dan Anderson.

Steinerman regrouped, thinking about the larger picture. There were close to six hundred thousand physicians including osteopathic physicians in the United States. What if the thousand-contract-thousand-year-minded Pyramids began to make inroads into other specialties? Just a nibble of a twenty-five thousand dollar a year "management" fee from a half-million practicing physicians by a few non-practicing M.D.s who no longer wanted to do rectal exams might be too big an untapped reservoir for the budding Pyramids and weasels to leave alone.

Every physician from every specialty might take note of the Pyramids, how easily the false prophets wrapped up one specialty, and how easily the fringe element might acquire the power in the future to skim a few dock fees from the endocrinologists or pediatricians. Stripminers without regulation might look at the sequoia forests of vascular surgery, gastroenterology, and the now vulnerable hospital-based radiology, anesthesiology, and pathology departments. Staff physicians might think twice about sitting there with their own thumbs up their asses the next time the stripminers attempt a "contract run" against their non-weasel, competent, self-managed, board-accredited, democratically-operated emergency department teams. It might be time to go to bat for those teams, not letting administration get fat on Beluga, and it might be time to think about the marketplace, how insidious the loose bantering of business terms has become, how "logical" it all seems, how the Goldman economic grand rounds makes pie-chart sense. All of medicine, physicians and patients alike, have some pretty high stakes in the success of unraveling the "suits." It's certainly in every physician's enlightened self-interest to loosen the noose of the crips and the bloods in emergency medicine "management" for "we have met the enemy and it is us."

While Steinerman thought, the phone suddenly rang, and both he and Eileen were stunned: it was Kensington. Steinerman had written to the thumbs up their asses six months ago challenging Kensington to a nationally televised debate on the situation in emergency medicine today. To his shock, the rather reckless American Academy took him up on his offer, and Kensington agreed to meet Steinerman on *Nighttime*. They would go at it, and show the American public once and for all that the "management" groups and weasels with their cronies in the Academy were proceeding with a fair, equitable system, leading to the advancement of emergency medical care, and were attracting the best of doctors who were staying in the field. Steinerman later learned Kensington, in a rare bit of bravado, acted on his own in accepting the offer from Tim Conley without consulting a single "suit," Kensington now suffering a new delusion about his role in emergency medicine.

Steinerman headed for New York. He had to agree to stay one week because they might be preempted for any fast-breaking news stories. Conley insisted they be live with at least one group in New York. On Tuesday the world was quiet, and at the scheduled hour, there he was, the Cat, Abraham David Steinerman, a long way from the General, hungry and ready to spring on his new prey.

Conley: So let me get this clear, Doctor. You're saying it is the marketplace that determines the quality of emergency medical care?

Kensington: That's exactly right, Tim, but what you're missing is the fact that the demand of consumers and their health-care dollars will sharpen the competitive edges of the groups, both large and small. The existence of the groups is actually one of the sources of pride of the American Academy of Emergency Physicians. You know, Tim, we're the only specialty that has the opportunity of having multistate corporations and their subsidiaries managing specialty health care in this country.

Conley: But, Doctor, that's exactly what Doctor Steinerman is saying is crippling the status of emergency medical care in the United States today. He says the groups and weasels are nothing but giant tapeworms, skimming exorbitant profits from the physicians working for them.

Kensington: Again, Tim, Doctor Steinerman underestimates the power of the marketplace. Look at it this way, Tim, let's say you put up ten thousand dollars to begin a business, or let's say you had put it into Apple Computer stock in 1979...

Steinerman watched with incredulity as Kensington kept making all of Steinerman's points. Kensington seemed to be on his side. Then it finally occurred to him, Kensington was simply dumb, a simple riboflavined mind at work.

"So that's why the American Academy loved him so much! Of course, with a dumb shit the likes of Kensington on the board of directors year after year, the thieves could keep on skimming forever. If the riboflavined idiot ever questioned them, they'd give him a mumbo-jumbo song and dance about voodoo economics, the birdbrain buying it every time." The cunning of the behind-the-scene powerbrokers of the American Academy never ceased to amaze Steinerman.

Goldman was aghast, watching Kensington spill the beans. Goldman was at first angry because he liked Kensington so much because of his overpowering neutrality. Then Goldman realized it, too. It wasn't his neutrality, it was his stupidity that he loved so much, his overpowering stupidity. He'd been a perfect president for the Academy and such a great audience for Goldman. Goldman sensed the end of an era, but immediately shoved the disagreeable thought deep into his subconscious. His anxiety, though, was rapidly building.

Kensington: ...and as you see, Tim, I'm just going to speak my mind.

"YOU DON'T HAVE A MIND," Goldman involuntarily screamed in his living room making Tahoe's house across the city shake like a seven point one on the Richter Scale. Goldman's outburst shocked even himself as he muttered, "Why didn't Kensington stay the potted plant we all knew and loved? Who the fuck let Kensington go on Nighttime anyway?"

Eileen Chen wondered herself why the Academy had let Kensington go on live television. She'd met Lyle, along with other "suits," when she chaired the emergency radiology committee, and she knew those well-spoken, savvy boys could give the large Cat a pretty difficult time.

She knew Kensington was quite the idiot the day he came over to the radiology department asking her "if she spoke Asian." Dr. Chen thought Kensington was subtly trying to ridicule her, but Kensington had a Hmong patient in the emergency room, and truly wondered if Dr. Chen could translate "Asian" for him. Goldman was certainly right about Kensington's mind.

Eileen became curious as to what a CAT scan of Kensington's brain would look like. The mountains and valleys of Kensington's cerebrum would certainly be heavy on the valleys, and there would be no Pikes Peaks, McKinleys, or Everests in that noodle. He had such a huge skull, though, his head could fill up the whole 27-inch Trinitron screen, but underneath that skull there would be a lot of valley, a lot of air, a lot of room. Kensington could probably survive a bout of meningitis, and maybe it was indeed the riboflavin that did this to him? Perhaps she should change Annie's vitamin regimen to none a day?

Eileen was certainly amused by Kensington's buffoonery tonight, and would get up early tomorrow because she didn't want to miss a word of commentary from any of the doctors in the morning coffee lounge.

Lyle watched in horror while Kensington continued:

Kensington: As one of our founding fathers, Doctor Norman Lyle, once said, "It's kind of like the Roman Catholic Church, you just obtain a few pennies from all the people."

Kensington was in a near babble at this point.

Kensington: ...and actually, Tim, Pyramid takes out only three hundred thousand dollars per year after expenses per hospital contract in Philadelphia for "management" fees, whereas the single "manager" in the past took over four hundred thousand dollars per hospital per year. When Pyramid took over the contracts, the income of the emergency physicians working there actually went up. So you see, Tim, the marketplace dictated that a larger group come into these hospitals and increase their quality of care, and quality, Tim, is after all, what we're all after (a little hint of a smile appeared on Kensington's face). The bigger the group the less they have to take out of each hospital to maintain or actually even increase the personal incomes of their corporate officers. It's simple arithmetic, Tim.

Kensington's broad grin was nine centimeters long, freezing on his face for a full fifteen seconds. Conley became concerned he had dislocated his jaw.

It was almost midnight when Conley was handed a note. The network agreed to go over since its president was watching, and knew this was going to be a big story. Conley himself was rather disturbed by these medical revelations, and felt a sudden panic flash through him as he thought of his wife and children. He declined to extend the interview, and after the show, nervously called his wife to make sure the family was o.k.

Lyle was physically ill at this point. He was nauseous, weak and dizzy. He felt febrile. He looked at his watch, hoping to God this nightmare would end. He became apoplectic, paralyzed with the thought of shame, national shame, knowing that he was wide open for the first set of investigations, the ones that would generate the most publicity and media scorn. This wasn't supposed to happen. He was supposed to have dignity, principle, honor, and be loved for all the work he did for the advancement of emergency medicine. Certainly his biography would win the Pulitzer Prize with knighthood shortly following, and he, Sir Norman, the final Canterbury tale, would sit ten feet tall in the saddle, riding through his long overdue, ticker-tape parade. He didn't sleep all night.

On the way to work he was passed by Adkins who was in town to speak at a pathology conference. Adkins shouted to Lyle at a red light, "Watch Nighttime last night?" He saw Lyle's face drop, and roared with laughter.

God, did Lyle hate that plowboy Adkins. Now the entire nation would be sneering at him. He entered the refuge of his office, gazing at the boat traffic in the Boston Harbor. He was safe now. This public-relations brush fire was nothing more than a challenge to greet enthusiastically, the whole untoward event now bringing out the fighter in him. Besides, it couldn't get any worse. His secretary Rene buzzed.

"A call on line one."

He braced, but wasn't prepared for this one. It was the Chancellor of the Stanford School of Medicine. He declined the Pyramid Chair of Emergency Medicine and the Pyramidology fellowship.

Goldman's son, Harvey, hadn't watched Nighttime that night. He was studying for the spring exams at Harvard. Harvey was a bright, kind-hearted student, and had recently been accepted to the Harvard Medical School. He was indeed the pride and joy of Goldman's life.

Goldman first got the call from his roommate that Harvey

had taken ill. He was seen at the student health service, and the attending physician sent him to the hospital, the Massachusetts General Hospital.

Harvey, however, knew better than to go to a public hospital staffed by interns and residents, even though it was a prestigious Harvard institution staffed by the finest interns and residents in the world. He'd heard his father extol the quality of the private hospitals, private doctors, in fact, anything private, and he insisted on being taken to Mount Zion.

Goldman panicked when Harvey's roommate told him, and he raced to his car, speeding to Zion. Nothing could be worse. Mount Zion was a Pyramid hospital, a marketplace hospital. Pyramid! Even one of his own hospitals would have been better! How could the student health physician let his son, the son of a physician, be taken to a Pyramid hospital? Surely they all knew! Goldman was stuck in traffic. He ran out to get a soda since he was dehydrated, covered in a cold, peculiarly lonely sweat.

It was 12:45 p.m. when Harvey Goldman was first seen by Doctor Monk. Monk noted a warm, actually hot, very ill-appearing white male in his late teens. The patient's ears were flushed with fever, his throat studded with pustules. Probably strep, Monk thought, and he had a brand new drug to give him. Harvey's eardrums were also bright red, but Monk never looked. His neck was stiff, lungs were clear, heart tones normal, and extremities unremarkable. When Monk pulled Harvey's right, lower eyelid down, he noted a peculiar, round red spot. It seemed vaguely familiar to him. He remembered a sick little girl from a small farm town in Southern Indiana with similar red spots and a high fever. He remembered how she got better with a cortisone cream. After all, he had never heard anything to the contrary. He dropped a solution of cortisone on the affected eye, and sent Harvey Goldman down for a chest x-ray.

During the hours Harvey waited for his turn, the bacteria in his spinal fluid doubled in number, and then doubled again, and then doubled, and doubled through a hundred new generations, and when his turn came, Harvey was too sick to stand for the chest film. When he was placed on the x-ray table he suffered a seizure. His body crashed to the floor with such a thunder he shattered his jaw and front row of teeth. The convulsion was so violent his wrist cracked as it involuntarily smashed into the bottom of the x-ray table. His tongue bled profusely from the first blow and the convulsive clenching of his jaw, chewing his tongue between the back molars. CODE BLUE was called while the radiologist watched in horror, the now petechiae-covered body thrashing about in an uncontrollable fit. The new emergency physician responded to the code first, as Monk's shift had ended over an hour ago, and he had gone home. The seizure ended, and the emergency physician, recognizing the seriousness of the situation, immediately transferred Harvey Goldman to the Massachusetts General Hospital. He lived another six hours in the intensive care unit.

He had an organ donation card in his wallet, but his brain was flattened, his kidneys laced with pus, his liver filled with micro-abscesses, and his adrenals had literally collapsed from the weight of the fulminate infection. He was cremated later the same day.

Several weeks later, Goldman returned to work, and after his decent interval, he'd resolved his anger, though not his grief. At first he planned to sue both Pyramid, Inc., and Monk, but that would surely reach the public eye like a mafia war of the families, and the cloak-and-dagger secrecy was of the utmost importance in preserving the "management" group system. He couldn't let petty factionalism destroy this system for which he had fought so long. The fact that he often used Monk to work for him would come out in court, and that would do Harvey no good. Besides, what the hell good would a million bucks do him now? He, like Lyle, couldn't even give it away. He was tired, and longingly wanted to return to the life of meetings in cities like New Orleans, telling anecdotal humorous stories, speaking proverbs from Satchel Paige and Yogi

Berra, exhorting emergency physicians to fight the big bad forces of government, and demanding short-sighted hospital administrators approve transcribing fees for effective chart wars. He wanted to hear the young residents wildly applaud him, and he wanted his reputation back, the one of the combination Mark Twain-Norman Rockwell dean of emergency medicine, the one he had so brilliantly and deceptively cultivated while the "scrubs" did all the heavy lifting. After all, he wasn't despised like Lyle, and besides, they needed him. Emergency medicine was beginning to question the value of people like himself.

"Those goddamned ingrates. I was the one who took them off the streets, giving them an agency to look up to. I placed them in jobs. They were so young and stupid, genetically too weak-willed and defective in moral character to even pick up the phone and call a hospital themselves. I was the one who created emergency medicine and just like that, I'm not going to give it back. I gave them that goofy, caretaker president for the Academy, and God damn it, I'll find them another one."

Goldman felt his juices flowing again. Besides they needed him, as several insurance companies began to question his high, six-figure income. Pretty soon they'd be questioning Lyle's multiple seven-figure income, asking, "Why are we giving these clowns millions, no, tens of millions of bucks every year to do a job unnecessary in every other specialty of medicine?" They wouldn't swallow the bullshit line of thinking as easily as Kensington. The government was also launching an investigation into shadowy group practices, and already an indicted hospital administrator in Des Moines was plea bargaining embezzlement charges, offering to testify on bribes against one of the Kansas-based "management" groups. The public needed Goldman to set things straight, the American Academy needed him, and now more than ever, Monk needed him.

Phoenix?

Yes.

I'm beginning to think you didn't make all of this up.

Oh?

I need to know about my community hospital down the street. I now have two small children, and am quite concerned there are no controls over emergency medicine other than the avarice of the bloods, crips, and weasels. Something's clearly out of kilter. The "suits" seem to have gotten something backwards. These physicians turned, as the American Academy calls them, "entrepreneurs," appear to be without any sense of decency, even within their own community?

That's my boys.

What should I ask, Phoenix?

Ask first if the emergency department is centrally managed by an absentee landlord.

Good start. What next?

Find out how much money leaves the local community for these "management" services.

Good. What next?

Look at any hefty donations any emergency medicine group or weasel is making in the community such as a local church, right-to-life-group, anti-defamation league, or YMCA.

Excellent. Continue.

Find out about weasels. How many physicians has your community hospital's emergency department gone through in the past ten years? Has only the director remained stable while the "scrubs" have "burned out" at an alarming rate? Find out, particularly, if any fine "scrubs" were picked up by other democratically-run local hospitals and kept there.

Good Phoenix. I'll pursue this, and will recruit other mothers, fathers, and grandparents in our neighborhood to press our hospital's board of directors for this information. It's our civic duty. Keep me posted.

I will.

CHAPTER TWENTY-FIVE

A MODEST PROPOSAL

"No lie can live forever."
—*Carlyle*

Philip Mahoney had just finished his last shift at Braintree Children's, and when he got home, Tahoe gave him a letter from Delorenzo, and played back a call from him on the answering machine.

Mahoney felt a certain camaraderie with Delorenzo since they were in the same residency program, having worked many nights together with the adrenalin flowing. Mahoney felt that certain foxhole loyalty of residents who'd worked together for three intensive years. In other words, he had to read Delorenzo's letter and return his phone call.

He wished he could have a couple of B & B's to get in the mood for Delorenzo's gloominess, but Delorenzo was surprisingly upbeat. He was writing the Model Emergency Medicine Contract for both hospitals and physicians. Delorenzo was coming through again. It was just like him, physician, humanist, and many times a torchbearer, to put together the formulation of fairness with no bullshit. Joe was calling and writing for feedback.

Dear Phil,

...and a national registry will be set up of all multistate, multiple-intrastate, and individual emergency medicine "management" corporations. The registry will contain the names, addresses, and phone numbers of any hospitals which in the past did not renew their contract with the "management" group, regardless of the stated reasons. This list needs to be submitted to the state health department of every state in which the group wishes to do business, even if it simply mails glossies to the hospital administrators.

By law, this list will also be submitted to every hospital administrator with which the group wishes to do business, fully apprising them of their past records, and this comprehensive list of non-renewed contracts has to go back to the inception of the groups, regardless of how many birthname changes, takeovers, buyouts, mergers or acquisitions its undergone. After all, no matter how many times people change their letterheads or business cards, a rose is still a rose, and we've yet to see the leopard with new spots. Stiff fines and prison terms will accompany any omissions or "oversights" on the list.

Immunity statutes would apply to all hospital administrators regarding libel and slander laws. Administrators would actually be encouraged to say exactly why they dropped the contract with any crip, blood, or weasel with which they chose not to continue. So if hospital A contacted hospital B to find out why hospital A dropped the crips, hospital A's administrator could say, "They promised me good docs, but gave me the shittiest group of misfits I've ever encountered." Regardless of what was said, a case of libel or slander could not be sustained in the courts, very similar to child abuse reporting statutes. We can't allow the "suits" to threaten hospital administrators with "intimidation lawsuits."

By federal law, a cap will be placed on true management fees, perhaps two to three dollars per patient visit. This may, in fact, solve everything. A formula would be devised allocating hard costs like malpractice and billings, and then a specific amount would be allowed for management fees. This would insure that the physician seeing a complicated case would receive the bulk of the fee or share the fee amongst a group of democratically-organized emergency physicians according to the Model Emergency Medicine Contract.

I would propose using the input from as many "scrubs" around the nation as we can. The era of the fantastically rich "managers" being generated by the nation's emergency departments would be ended for good. It's high time for a new order to rise, grounding the high fliers. The collapse of their empires will be the greatest thing for the specialty of emergency medicine since the accreditation board was approved.

You see, Phil, the way emergency medicine has existed would be analogous to saying Yellowstone is a national park, but there will be no regulations. We all know pretty soon the Snake River would be fished out and following that, the osprey and eagles would die off. Poachers would eliminate the elk herds in a matter of a few years, and timber companies would eliminate the danger of forest fires forever. This is the way the landscape of emergency medicine has been pillaged over the past two decades, and the reason is the nonexistent set of rules. It's amazing to me the extent of the theft. I now agree with you and Abe Steinerman that the lack of regulation has spawned this perverse situation existing today which creates entry barriers to new physicians.

The American Academy will obviously fight tooth

> and nail against a mandatory, model contract for both hospitals and physicians, and will insist upon putting another coat of paint on the outhouse, giving a stripped-down version of lip-service reform, providing giant loopholes for the "suits." Reform then, must proceed through the imposition of federal regulations on emergency medicine "management."
>
> We clinical doctors need to risk a little regulatory action to annihilate deceptive practices, rather than accept yet another Academy-approved self-enrichment scheme. There's really no other way to realize reform since we "scrubs" have lost control of the Academy, and that group of Pinocchios sure as hell aren't working for us. They're also going to give us that old ridiculous poppycock that a little regulation to unload these white elephants of emergency medicine will lead to the wholesale nationalization of all of medicine. The crips, bloods, and weasels have had quite a grip on emergency medicine for over two decades, and we aren't going to take away their easy sumptuous lifestyles or their gigantic cash cows too easily. But if we want to put a little perestroika into emergency medicine, we're going to have to sweep out the politburo along with their acolytes in the Academy. We may not be able to do it overnight, but I'm quite hopeful, Phil, we can make progress on a reform initiative in an incredibly short period of time.

Mahoney was feeling a certain surge of elation and pride as well as a little guilt. "What a bad time to be leaving emergency medicine," he thought. "With Delorenzo on the launching pad, the 'scrubs' might be able to pull it off, and pull it off with incredible velocity." Mahoney continued to read while Tahoe noticed the smile on his face grow broader.

> ...and we need to eliminate those noncompete

clauses, and holster the legal firepower of the "suits." The noncompete clauses should fall like the Berlin Wall, with a federal law as an effective antidote against them. Otherwise, we'll continue to see our friends roughed up by the high handed. We've already lost too many good physicians who initially had vague career goals in mind. We now have to stem the exodus of some of the best and brightest in our specialty.

It's absurd to think if you work in an emergency department, especially in a large city, that there are numerous options for the practicing doctor. I remember when Pyramid stole my contract at Good Sam, how I tried to joke with my docs, telling them, "I've got a pretty limited disposition option for you all." I had to give them their one way ticket to Palookaville. It is clearly a de facto restraint of trade to force the emergency physician to work for the same "management" group in the same area for the rest of time. It's imperative to give the "scrubs" the level playing field they need and deserve. After two years, retroactive from the passage of the bill, a group of physicians can elect whether to self-manage, contract with another group, or stay with the same group. This doesn't mean the physician has to pack his or her bags, call Bekins, pluck their kids out of grade school, and leave for two years. States can be more liberal, if they chose, perhaps limiting it to one year. This will rattle the future fortunes of the "suits," but it will require a grass roots movement of "scrubs" and consumers to pass.

But, Phil, we can do it. It will certainly be a bloodied event, but decolonization of the nation's emergency departments is an inevitability, and the sooner we get this off the starting blocks the better. There's no doubt in my mind there is sufficient willpower and courage within the "scrubs" to remove those who so easily seized untold wealth. Our entire specialty is marred by these destroyers of good medical care.

We are also going to require a close federal court monitorship of this egregious gambit of buying and selling emergency medicine contracts, an obscene practice of which I've recently become aware.

Phil, don't blame our teachers for this either. They were obviously unaware of what was going on. Remember, Phil, our teachers gave us a gift, a gift that cannot be silenced, even by the weight of the present leadership of the American Academy of Emergency Physicians.

The American Academy has long since abandoned its watchdog role, and we have every reason to believe it will deliberately sit on these recommendations, allowing further unfair diversion of physicians' incomes to the contract holders. We need to put the harsh spotlight on this entire field ourselves with a new organization.

We need to inform Democrats and Republicans alike of the *On The Waterfront* maneuverings and injustices, the sheer gangsterism that has so conventionally evolved under the auspices of the "Founders" and the Academy of Emergency Physicians. Their uncooked corporate books have to be exposed to a bipartisan congressional hearing, their IRS returns verified, and if anyone lies, they need to serve hard time. Institutionalized perjury, the underpinning of the American Academy, has to be exposed to the judiciary, and the same judiciary that couldn't be stopped in Watergate or Iranscam can steamroller over the Emergi-RICH.

Also the public, Mr. and Mrs. John Q., can decide if it makes sense for the "manager" of a single group to make more than the physician seeing their child. Mr.

and Mrs. John Q. can decide if fifty-one dollars of their one-hundred-dollar fee should go to the contract holder, twenty for expenses, and twenty-nine to the physician who treats their child. They, not the American Academy, who feels this is a perfect formulation, can decide the fee distribution. The Q's can tell Travelers, Medicare, and Blue Cross how to distribute the fee, and tell all practicing emergency physicians to get off their duff, form a new organization, and end their collective victimization, for themselves, and most importantly, for the Mary G.'s and Jennys everywhere, and to end forever the rape of emergency medicine.

Sincerely,

Joe

MAHONEY'S COMMANDMENTS OF EMERGENCY MEDICINE

The more states a physician is licensed in, the more incompetent he usually is.

Corollary one: Multi-licensed incompetent physicians are equally incompetent in all states in which they work.

There's a bigger fortuna in emergency medicine "management" than there is in shit.

The competence of physicians working in an emergency department is inversely proportional to the number of promotional "products" and "services" merchandised by the emergency medicine "management" group.

The crips and the bloods with the most extensive "quality assurance" programs assure the lowest-quality physicians.

The more money and time a "suit" spends on risk management, the more he increases the risk.

Taking a sick child to a non-owner-occupied "doc in the box" is a form of child abuse.

Corollary one: Always ask about the owner of a "doc in the box."

"Suits" of whatever stripe should not run for public office at any level.

"The business of America is business." (Uncle Calvin)

Corollary One: The business of organized emergency

medicine is business.

The smaller the child the larger the cast.

Always err on the side of treatment.

Never say OOPS, always say THERE.

The more pressing the emergency, the more likely the suction machine will fail.

One of the reasons for medical protocol is bias.

and,

“The secret of caring for the patient is to care for the patient.”